T0178616

Disruptive Cooperation in Digital Health

Jody Ranck
Editor

Disruptive Cooperation in Digital Health

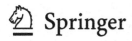 Springer

Editor
Jody Ranck
HealthBank
Chevy Chase, MD
USA

ISBN 978-3-319-82232-7   ISBN 978-3-319-40980-1   (eBook)
DOI 10.1007/978-3-319-40980-1

Printed on acid-free paper

This Springer imprint is published by Springer Nature
The registered company is Springer International Publishing AG Switzerland

Acknowlegments

We would like to acknowledge the generous contributions from Dr. Jonathan Javitt and the Blue Cross Blue Shield Foundation of California and their assistance in making this book possible.

Contents

Chapter 1
Disruptive Cooperation: Innovation for Health's Wicked Problems

Jody Ranck

Healthcare systems are in transition worldwide and are feeling the pressure to deliver better outcomes at lower costs. By now, most readers will have heard the statistics. The USA has the most expensive healthcare system in the world based on per capita spending, yet we rank 37th in the world in health outcomes according to the World Health Organization. If we break this down, the numbers are even more sobering. On an annual basis, the WHO estimates that the US infant mortality rate ranks even lower in the global rankings and we are frequently hovering in the 40s for adult female mortality.[1] This is a system that consumes approximately $2.6 trillion annually, nearly 20 % of GDP. Just to give you an idea of what these numbers mean—this amount is the equivalent of the sixth largest economy on the planet. The challenges to the healthcare system are only growing. In many European and middle-income countries, we find aging populations, prolonged financial crises, and growing health disparities—all demand new solutions and a renewed engagement with health care that can rise above the political polemics. China will see over 10,000 villages with very few residents under 70 years of age in the next decade and will need to find new ways to deliver health care to this aging population. We can no longer afford to have a healthcare system become such a drain on the economy without delivering results in terms of population health outcomes. Rethinking the delivery of health care has become both a sustainable economics question and a public health imperative. For many, the arrival of digital health technologies was going to be the answer to the many challenges

---

[1]Christopher Murray and Julio Frenk. N Engl J Med 2010; Ranking 37th—Measuring the Performance of the US Healthcare System. 362:98–99.

J. Ranck (✉)
Health Bank, Ranck Consulting, Ram Group, Washington, D.C., USA
e-mail: jody@ranckconsulting.com

© Springer International Publishing Switzerland 2016
J. Ranck (ed.), *Disruptive Cooperation in Digital Health*,
DOI 10.1007/978-3-319-40980-1_1

listed above. We argue that they are a necessary part of the solution, but the *social dimensions of innovation are neglected. Cooperation is going to be the key driver to realize the triple aim of lower costs, better outcomes, and population health*. Innovation needs to move beyond technology to new ways of thinking about co-creation, co-innovation, the commons, and public goods. These can also drive sustainable business success that also creates healthier populations.

This is not merely a technological issue but demands new ways of thinking about organizational change and the place of technology in these new organizational forms. New business models with complex value chains and ecosystems of stakeholders are needed to address health care's "wicked problems" where no one-off, single-point solution will fix health care's woes. The problems are multidimensional and go well beyond medical care systems—health outcomes are a window into how societies work; there is a health production function that spans social status, environmental drivers, individual choices, and behaviors, as well as the functioning of health systems and our genetics. Precision medicine will need to address the multicausal nature of health outcomes and not just focus on genetics. Wicked problems cannot be "fixed" by single, one-off solutions but require the leadership to marshal together an ecosystem approach and fresh ways of thinking about **designing health systems for desired outcomes**. Health care has yet to succeed in producing a platform that can tie together new business models and services in the manner we have seen Apple, Google, Microsoft, or Facebook. Yet new technologies such as Blockchain may enable new business models and practices for sharing data beyond the data silos that dominate in the present. The notion of a platform that enables new business models and sharing of data across vendors, patients, and providers, and different health systems is becoming an imperative. A major theme of this book is that health care is becoming part of a growing digital service economy, and many lessons on how to build complex digital solutions can come from approaches *informed by design and cooperative business models found in other sectors*. If we build more cooperative business models with the scale and scope to address the complexities of today's challenges, we can begin to think about transforming our health systems to respond to actual needs. Here, we are talking about disruption in the following way. Cooperation means utilizing the tools of co-innovation with communities, patients, and other companies and across competitors, payers, and providers. New technologies slapped on old ways of doing business based on data capture, and creating silos has a limited shelf-life. Competitors, if they think beyond short-term gains, may find that sharing data can enable new business models to be derived from these data that are better capable of improving outcomes. Therefore, the concept of the commons is important. Interoperability does apply not only to data standards but also to organizational interoperability and business practices.

Let us face it, there is an entire health economy that benefits from the dysfunction we find in health systems, and these antiquated business models are slow to change. They will not be replaced overnight, but new entrants into the healthcare space cooperating with more forward thinking health enterprises could prove to be as powerful a motivator to system change as policy initiatives. From a policy perspective, the old guard that benefited from the sickness economy will need to be de-incentivized, and this includes some of the largest players in health technology whose antiquated business models based on data capture rather than sharing data for the common good should be incentivized into extinction or change their ways, quite frankly. They have become a public health problem as much as they represent a Faustian bargain for large hospitals and providers. Health care is becoming another digital service, which does not mean we have to lose the human component. But leveraging the massive amounts of data for better individual and population health outcomes will not be accomplished via many of the traditional business models. There is a true (r)evolution in meaning and how we think about healthcare delivery. Digital hospitals will have a very different approach that may overlap with current models but will need to extend into communities and homes, for example. Organizational interoperability will count as much as technological interoperability to improve the quality and scalability of health services. In the final days of writing this book, we saw the launching of new partnerships on Blockchain and health care when two technology companies, Gem and Philips, launched a joint venture with a call to bring other Blockchain and health technology companies together. We want to encourage initiatives like this and feel that Blockchain and cooperation could, in the long haul, make a significant contribution to better health systems.

The Business Case

A tipping point has been reached where the incentives that support the underlying healthcare business model have begun to change—and it has begun already to tilt ever so slightly toward a more prevention-oriented system from the sickness economy that has become unsustainable. Value-based care is a systemic driver that is enabling new business models for prevention. To put it in more human terms, wouldn't it be better to offer a diabetic better preventive care to the tune of $7000–10,000 than to pay $65,000 to amputate a foot due to lack of preventive care? We have both technological and non-technological solutions to avoid this type of system failure, but all too often the incentives and coordination of care are not there to prevent these failures. Who gets rewarded for cooperating and coordinating care? New payment mechanisms under value-based care have begun to reward healthcare providers who do a better job of coordinating care and reducing hospital admissions. While this is the beginning, we think much more intellectual and policy work needs to be done to marshal technologies, business practices, and platforms to succeed. We have written this book to offer hope and show that there are solutions to many of the problems we face. We are living in a historical moment of rapid technological change, and the coming years will demand a great deal of more collaboration across the public and private sectors, between patients and clinicians, public health, and medicine. The exciting thing is that many of the technologies we will write about in this book have already demonstrated their transformative potential for new forms of cooperation and business models in other sectors of the economy. **The innovation we are going to discuss in this book is not just a story about new gadgets and devices, however. We discuss devices and technologies but are making a call for more efforts that demonstrate a focus on cooperation and co-creation can change the way we deliver health care and reconfigure systems to more patient-centric care.**

The technological shift that is beginning to transform our healthcare system, albeit slowly, is different from many of the technological shifts of the past due to a number of concurrent factors:

- The key driver is the growth of mobile phone access, particularly for smartphones in the past 4–5 years, and the computing power embodied by these devices will make them central devices for patients to manage conditions in the coming years.
- We may have reached a tipping point where the cost of health care is viewed as unsustainable in the eyes of all stakeholders across the healthcare value chain.
- Low-cost sensors are becoming quasi-ubiquitous and will continue to grow for the foreseeable future and enable the development of a "health Internet of Things" that includes the medical home, more wired hospitals, and environmental sensors. A great deal of policy innovation is required to minimize the risks associated with these technologies and optimize system transformation. These also carry with them risks and fears of surveillance that will demand both technology innovation and policy innovation.
- The tools that enable us to make sense of the data collected across the ecosystem have begun to scale in ways that can possibly keep pace with the growth in data and knowledge across the health sciences. Yet precision medicine has a long way to go to bridge the gap between the technology infrastructure used in genomics (-omics in general) and the health IT infrastructure that will render these data useful to clinicians and patients.
- Many-to-many platforms as embodied in social media are empowering patients, innovators, and community-based groups to share insights and build communities of interest around health issues. How can we mobilize citizens and civil society to push for the necessary policy and technological changes that have not been effective so far in catalyzing transformational change?
- Governments have discovered new mechanisms to unlock health data and build platforms for individuals and innovators to build new products and services that can address some of the inefficiencies, information asymmetries, and gaps in services that exist in our current fragmented system of care. The time is ripe to take lessons from the experiments to date and build strategies that can leverage these platforms even more with an eye toward transformational change of health systems. Policies need to catch up to technology and cultural shifts so that cloud computing can be better leveraged and incentives for good governance in place. Blockchain growth will only further the need for policy innovations as the capabilities of a distributed, cryptographic ledger enable distributed, autonomous corporations and may render insurance models as we know them in the present, archaic.

What is emerging is more than a one-off technology shift but a new ecosystem of technologies and even policy frameworks that will steadily transform the health-care system over the next decade. *The algorithmic revolution is beginning to transform health care.*

We begin with many of the challenges in the health system, but our goal is to offer some insights into some of the potential directions the system will go in the coming decade. This does not mean that technology has all of the answers for technological solutions also require social, cultural, and political changes to bring about the necessary changes. Despite the challenging political and economic realities in which we find ourselves at the moment, we still have a tremendous opportunity to create a better healthcare system. This is going to be a long-term process, not a simple matter of a single shot at health reform by any single administration, but a long-term transformation of health systems and a revolution in what health and health care *mean* in a digital world. Over the past several years, we have witnessed a dramatic growth in wireless technologies that offer the promise of extending the reach of our healthcare system while offering many early-stage solutions that hold the promise of saving money and lives. For many, this may sound like another round of hype from the technology sector promising riches and futuristic marvels that rarely materialize, except for the few. Many readers have undoubtedly heard this before with genomics and biotechnology from the late 1980s to the present. Biotechnologies would offer a myriad of wonder cures for cancer, chronic diseases, and a host of other diseases. One to two decades later, we have certainly seen many advances in the time and costs it takes to sequence a human genome and there are many new therapies on the market that can save or extend lives. But for the average patient, the "revolution" often appears lacking. Drugs that cost over $100,000 per year and may extend a life 6–12 months have not reached the bar for counting as transformational unless they have widespread access and dramatically improved outcomes. The biotech revolution has been uneven and has not addressed the fundamental structural problems in our healthcare system. In fact, the prices for biologicals can contribute to pressure on healthcare prices. Digital health technologies have the capacity to bring down the cost of clinical trials and ultimately the price of new drug entities. Innovations, if they are worthy of the label, will need to be measured by their capacity to offer better care to more people at a lower price. Precision medicine will need to evolve beyond genomics to include environmental, social, and behavioral drivers of health outcomes to have the efficacy it promises. Doing this will require ways of building new data commons and the ability to push analytics insights to the point of care and into the home. At present, this is a very challenging order and the health information technology infrastructure is poorly prepared despite marketing rhetoric to the contrary.

The growth in wireless health and health IT in general, if coupled with the right mix of organizational change across the health system, could play a major role in reducing inefficiencies and improving the overall quality of care if we make the right policy decisions and build a collaborative market for these innovations in the coming years. Competition is an important part of what drives innovation in health care but not the only dynamic that matters. Just throwing technology at health issues and calling it "disruptive" is beginning to lose its luster.

We are in the early days of the wireless health era, but the impact is already visible. Many readers will have already experimented with an app for monitoring their diet, fitness, or a chronic condition such as diabetes. Fitbits have become ubiquitous but are hardly the answer for solving chronic disease self-care. You may have noticed a change in the past one or two years when you entered your doctor's office and encountered an electronic health record (EHR) for the first time, unless you have been getting your health care from one of the early adopters who implemented EHRs years ago. Many of you may belong to an online patient group or social network where you can share experiences of managing a chronic condition or get involved with a health campaign. Some innovations are more subtle, an app that lets you see the air pollution levels in your neighborhood and determines who contributes to pollution levels in your zip code, for example. Several years ago, having the power in your hand to "see" this information would have been unimaginable. Today, we can use the camera in our cell phones to get a reading of your heart rate and the author is involved with a company that will soon have sensors on the market that offer a full EKG plus several other biometric measures and the sensor can be manufactured for pennies. Hackathons and innovation challenges are proliferating around the world for solutions that can address the chronic disease epidemic or the health challenges of cities. One interesting example is an innovation challenge sponsored by Qualcomm to develop a "health tricorder" that can measure all of your vital signs with a mobile device. These are just some of the examples of the changes that are happening that we will document in the chapters that follow.

We would like to take you a journey across the healthcare system and provide the reader with insights into what the future of the health care could look like in the coming years if we get things right this time around. On many of these fronts, there is no consensus on the best path forward and the contributors to this book have a strong interest in focusing on new approaches to building platforms that can scale and create ecosystems and new business models focused on the triple aim.

How (un)Healthy Are We?

Before we dive into the technology innovations that concern us, we will take a brief detour into the problems with the US healthcare system. This will provide the context for the unmet needs and challenges for which entrepreneurs are actively developing solutions. We will learn how specific chronic diseases and relatively small numbers of poorly managed conditions contribute to substantial financial costs that we all pay for through higher health insurance premiums and other "taxes." Social innovation that can bring about policy innovations and organizational change will need to accompany the technologies if we are to drive disruptive change. One of the lessons that the rise of social networking platforms and data analytics are demonstrating is that health outcomes are often tied to the social networks and communities in which we inhabit. Mobile phones, we will learn, are helping us to understand the social dynamics of chronic diseases beyond the issue of individual choice. Health is a profoundly social issue, and we are only in the early days of leveraging "social technologies" such as the Web and mobile to produce healthier communities. Data mining, when done in an ethical manner, can uncover hidden patterns that may not be observable to the clinical gaze. We will examine research that illustrates the connections between the relative health status of our social networks and one's risk of being obese or eventually receiving a diabetes diagnosis. This is important to keep in mind as we look at the statistics below.

The Challenge of Chronic Diseases

We live in a society that is aging. The antibiotic revolution that played a dramatic role in extending life spans after World War II has played a major role in helping to shape the demographic profile of the US population. In 1910, about the time that the architecture of our current medical system was being formed, the percentage of Americans 60 or over was nearly 7 %. By 2020, the percentage of Americans over 60 is projected to be over 20 %.[2] Many countries such as Italy and Japan[3] are facing severe shortages of caregivers given the demographics of aging that leave a gap in the health workforce that aging in place technologies can help fill. This shift alone translates into an increase in chronic diseases that accompany the aging process. In addition, we have a serious problem in the USA and elsewhere with many suffering from chronic conditions at a younger age. *Chronic obstructive pulmonary disease (COPD) alone will cost $4.8 trillion globally by 2030.*[4] Childhood obesity rates have skyrocketed as our food system and lifestyles have shifted. When we take a look at the numbers below, the challenge of chronic diseases will appear daunting. But the fact is that most chronic diseases are preventable. It is not too late to change the trends and forecasts if we take can target our energies and resources to bring incentives and policies in alignment around what should be done rather than continue to support the policies and incentives that have created the problems in the first place. Below are some statistics to illustrate just how serious a problem we are confronting and some of the economic statistics associated with chronic diseases are staggering:

---

[2]http://www.aoa.gov/aoaroot/aging_statistics/index.aspx.

[3]http://www3.weforum.org/docs/WEF_Harvard_HE_GlobalEconomicBurdenNon CommunicableDiseases_2011.pdf.

[4]http://www3.weforum.org/docs/WEF_Harvard_HE_GlobalEconomicBurdenNon CommunicableDiseases_2011.pdf.

- More than 67 % of baby boomers have one or more chronic diseases.[5]
- More than 109 million Americans have at least one of the seven main chronic diseases such as diabetes, heart disease, cancer, or arthritis totaling over 162 million cases.
- The total economic impact of chronic diseases accounts for over $1.3 trillion annually.
- Chronic diseases account for $1.1 in lost productivity and $227 billion for treating these conditions.
- At the current rate, it is projected that we will see a 42 % increase in chronic conditions by 2023 that will contribute to an economic loss of $4.2 trillion annually.
- Even modest improvements in prevention and treatment could reduce these costs by up to 42 %.
- Prevention alone could reduce chronic disease rates by 27 % and save $1.1 trillion and save $218 billion that would have gone to the cost of treatment. The net result would be a $905 billion increase in GDP.
- 23 million Americans have asthma, resulting in over 500,000 hospitalizations per year, many preventable.
- One in ten people in the USA has diabetes, and approximately 350 million individuals worldwide have been diagnosed with the condition.
- Either over 50 % of prescriptions for drugs are left unfilled or patients do not adhere to the prescribed regimen properly.
- Readmissions after acute care costs Medicare $12 billion annually and across all taxpayers approximately $25 billion annually.[6]
- Nearly 75 %, or approximately $1.7 trillion, of all health spending in the USA per year is linked to chronic heart failure, chronic obstructive pulmonary disorder, and diabetes.[7]
- While the attention has been on the "diabesity epidemic" in the USA, by 2030 the growth in disease rates in middle-income countries will be substantial given current trajectories.

Seventy percent of all deaths are caused by chronic diseases with heart disease, cancer, and stroke accounting for half of all causes of mortality. Pragmatic measures we can use to cut costs. Health care has its own version of a 1 % crisis.[8] Currently, the top 1 % of healthcare users consume about 21.8 % of all health expenditures and the top 5 % of users consume *over 50 % of the overall health*

---

[5]2010 Survey of Health Consumers: Key findings, strategic implications. Deloitte Center for Health Solutions, May 2010.

[6]See the Institute for Healthcare Improvement, State Action on Avoidable Readmissions program: http://www.ihi.org/offerings/initiatives/staar/Pages/default.aspx.

[7]Stachura, M. and Khasanshina, E. (2007). Tele-homecare and Remote Monitoring: An Outcomes Review (Advamed 2007). Available: http://www.advamed.org.

[8]http://meps.ahrq.gov/mepsweb/data_files/publications/st354/stat354.shtml.

expenditures.[9] Many of the factors that drive these utilization rates are social. We often hear now that your zip code tells us more about your health than your genetic code. If we can move the dial in these segments of the population alone by helping them to become healthier before they fall ill with expensive acute conditions, we can make a significant dent in the waste that our healthcare system produces. Just to give the reader an idea of how fast the chronic disease epidemic is growing, we can look at the data for 2000 when we had approximately 125 million suffering from chronic diseases. If we look ahead to 2020, it is projected that 157 million will suffer from at least one chronic disease. Our current system is too expensive to treat and manage all of the cases in a sustainable way over the life course of every patient. Many middle-income countries will have to simultaneously deal with a large burden of infectious diseases as well as growing chronic disease rates, making the need for health system transformation even stronger. The underlying economic model of care combined with the structure of the healthcare system has rewarded payment for rendering of services (fee-for-service model) versus paying for generating good health outcomes. This is beginning to change, and we will need to go farther to reign in costs in the coming years. Digital health solutions will be critical tools for health system stakeholders to succeed in the coming value-driven health economy that will increasingly emphasize prevention and keeping people out of hospitals.

The past system of rewards made keeping people out of hospitals a challenge. In 2007, the Medicare Payment Advisory Committee studied the economics of hospital readmissions for chronic diseases and found that inadequately handling the discharge of patients from the hospital resulted in increased expenditures for readmissions of 17.6 % higher to the tune of $15 billion annually. Seventy-five percent of these readmissions were deemed preventable.[10] A large number of these preventable readmissions can be readily resolved through wireless technologies combined with new case management systems. These numbers do not even reflect the toll of readmissions on families and caregivers. As we will see later, the economic costs of caregiving have become a major issue in the USA and many readers will be acutely aware of the sacrifices they make in time and income managing the health care of a sick family member or friend.

The sheer complexity of treating people with multiple chronic diseases is a challenge as well. Most treatment guidelines focus on a single disease, and many risk models used to manage patient populations are also based on single or tightly linked conditions. As we age and have to manage multiple conditions, some of the guidelines may actually contradict one another. Osteoporosis may demand more weight-bearing exercise, for example, while guidelines for some diabetics may have the patient avoid weight-bearing exercise. This is where personalized medicine based on a large amount of data from the medical literature combined with one's own personal health data can offer potentially better, more customized

---

[9]http://www.nccor.org/downloads/Understanding%20US%20Health%20Care%20Spending.pdf.

[10]http://www.himss.org/content/files/ControlReadmissionsTechnology.pdf.

treatment patterns for those suffering from a number of conditions and risk factors. For many chronic diseases, the solution is a shift in lifestyle choices such as diet and exercise but often things such as work, unsafe neighborhoods, and income levels get in the way. Fortunately, many of the tools used in wireless health can also help patients with social supports, building community coalitions, and other forms of social safety nets. We will explore how digital health solutions can take innovative community-level public health programs such as the healthy cities/communities initiative that married city planning and public health in the 1980s and reinvigorate these approaches in ways that can tie individual self-care to population health. One of the greatest challenges to realizing the vision of personalized medicine is the sheer capacity of health IT systems to integrate other types of data from beyond the clinic such as genomic data and patient-generated data. In the coming years, better integration of data, as well as user-friendly tools that provide insights to patients and providers, will be needed so that these data can be acted upon.

Aging in Place and Digital Health

The experience of aging is changing as well. We are living longer, and while many baby boomers live active lifestyles, the number of boomers and those more senior living with multiple chronic diseases is growing. A more mobile population means that it has become challenging for families to take care of a parent with dementia, for example, who may live in a distant city. Managing an aging population is becoming an important social and political issue in our financially challenged times. How can we keep people well throughout their twilight years so that they can continue to lead active and productive lives? There is a growing interest in how to rethink aging and to develop new roles for active seniors. This is an approach that is gaining in importance as many OECD countries face potential trade-offs in the context of the global financial crisis. Health systems can focus on a zero-sum game between the old and young and cut services for the elderly, or take a more holistic view and examine how to use new technologies that enable more active "silver years" and the opportunities this creates. Organizations like the International Longevity Centre are attempting to move beyond the zero-sum mind-set and explore new roles in the voluntary sector for those on pensions or in retirement. Prevention and well-being programs are increasingly emphasized throughout the life course so that the chronic disease burden described above can be attenuated later in life. The life course approach to aging can help us move beyond the zero sum, blame the elderly for bankrupting the system approach, and take a more holistic approach that focuses on lifestyles and behavioral interventions that can reduce chronic disease burdens. Mobiles and remote monitoring can play a very important role in facilitating behavioral changes, even later in life, that can reduce chronic disease burdens as well as making communities more livable for the elderly.

Some readers may balk at the thought of the elderly being mass users of technologies to manage their health conditions. There are several reasons to reconsider preconceived notions about technology and the elderly. First, it is time to take a long-term view of the problem over the next 10–20 years and plan ahead—the past may not be a good indicator of what the experience of aging will be like in 2015. The baby boomer generation has already adopted mobile technologies over the past decade and will likely continue to integrate many of these devices into their lifestyles if the technologies help improve their livelihoods. Second, many mobile technologies are designed specifically for aging patients who may have experienced diminishing dexterity, eyesight, and a number of other capacities. Many remote monitoring sensors will be worn in one's clothing and require little manipulation. Most signs are pointing to the fact that baby boomers are going to push for a very different experience of aging from their parents, and technology will play a big part in this transformation. In fact, aging technologies are becoming a major business opportunity for entrepreneurs looking beyond the newest, hippest device for the 18- to 32-year-old crowd.

Already, a number of wireless solutions are available to address conditions of aging. Unsafe wandering of patients with Alzheimer's increases the risk of injury and death. We can use sensors to monitor the location of those suffering from dementia and Alzheimer's. Falls are another major condition where wireless devices can help. According to the CDC, the economic burden of falls among the elderly will cost the US healthcare system over $50 billion and nearly 15,000 die per year from falls.[11] Wireless health solutions have been developed to monitor and even prevent falls through technologies such as smart slippers that monitor movements in the house.[12] The "Patient-Centered Medical Home" has proven to be a far more medically effective and cost-efficient way to manage many conditions associated with aging and is facilitated by telehealth and machine-to-machine (M2M) solutions that facilitate the access to a nurse or medical provider in one's home. This is an exciting area of work in the wireless health arena that can fundamentally change the way we experience aging—aging at home rather than in nursing homes. In Japan, the postal service realized that the Internet was resulting in far less mail needing to be delivered, so they equipped postal workers with tablet computers to monitor checkups on the elderly. This type of thinking needs more support and cross-fertilization with technologists, social scientists, and policy-makers along with an engaged citizenry to translate small changes into macro-outcomes.

Wearable technologies that were initially developed for the military and first responders are now playing a role in remote care. Armed with sensors that can detect heart rates, respiration rates, location, and even posture, these technologies will be deployed across the spectrum from fitness to aging. Already, we see the

---

[11]http://www.cdc.gov/homeandrecreationalsafety/Falls/data.html.

[12]http://mobihealthnews.com/5675/att-develops-smart-slippers-for-fall-prevention/.

use of sensors in elite European soccer matches and can see in real time the distance run by players, their velocity, temperature, and heart rates. These same tools can be used to get patients out of hospitals sooner and avoid the risk of hospital-acquired infections. Wearables and remote sensors can also be configured to send data to one's caregivers and not just your physician. There effects could be widely felt in the underlying economics of caregiving that has become a major challenge for many families in the USA with aging and sick relatives.

Aging and chronic diseases are not only issues for the afflicted alone. Taking care of sick relatives and friends can be a very costly and time-consuming commitment for approximately 29 % of the US population.[13] The economics of caregiving illustrate how the breakdown in our health system is taking a toll on households who provide approximately $375 billion annually in uncompensated care (ibid). That is twice as much than is spent on nursing home services and home care. Medical bills cause more than 50 % of bankruptcies in the USA. The average Medicare beneficiary pays an estimated $45,000 out of pocket for home care expenses each year.[14] According to the study cited above, more than 34 million individuals are providing care to another family member. Valuated at $10 per hour, this care amounts to more than $350 billion annually. In countries where extended families live together, the dynamics may be a bit different from the US context, but there are certainly tools that can help ease the burden globally for caregivers. Clearly, people need solutions that can facilitate and coordinate caregiving and offer better care at a lower cost. Even if you are perfectly healthy, the gaps in the healthcare system can have a profound effect on your quality of life. Remote monitoring and wearable technologies can play a role in enabling safer and more meaningful aging in place, but so far aging has been a relatively untapped market for many wearables makers who focus on the young and fit.

Waste and Inefficiencies

In 2012, the Institute of Medicine released a major report on the state of the US healthcare system.[15] The report highlights the coming perfect storm of dramatic growth in medical knowledge coming up against the growing disease burden and a system ill-equipped to handle the dual challenge of information overload and disease burden. It is easy to blame all of the problems surrounding our system on a single scapegoat—drug companies charging too much, government waste and paperwork, fragmentation of providers, and so on. In reality, there are problems

---

[13]Caregiving in the United States, 2009. National Alliance for Caregiving and the AARP.

[14]Valuing the Invaluable: A New Look at the Economic Value of Family Caregiving. AARP Public Policy Institute, 2007.

[15]Institute of Medicine, 2012. Best Care at a Lower Cost: The Path to Continuously Learning Healthcare in America.

throughout the system that stem from the incentives for payment, lack of a data-driven system, and silos that make getting the right information at the right time to the right person next to impossible, to the rising cost of clinical trials and beyond. One of the problems that may not be appreciated by the general public is the challenge of our successes in science and research. The sheer volume of knowledge and data produced by the health and medical sciences is now impossible to fully comprehend by any single medical or health professional. What we are learning is that it is one thing to generate vast amount of medical data and quite another to actually integrate the data into clinical care.

The IOM report suggests that it would take 21 h per day for primary care physicians to provide all of the recommended care for acute, preventive, and chronic care for management needs. In addition to clinical care and keeping up with the latest medical science, physicians spend approximately 30 % of their time on administrative work that has become increasingly complex as the system has grown. It should come as no wonder then that patient care is often fragmented as the patient moves from a primary care provider to specialists. Most often, the tools that we need to coordinate and assist physicians to manage their workflows either have not existed or have not be up to the task at hand. The bottlenecks listed here also play a role in increasing medical errors. Several years ago, the IOM studied the problem of medical errors and determined that 100,000 lives per year are lost due to preventable errors.

In order to provide the highest quality of care, clinicians increasingly need tools that can help them keep up with the rapid rate of growth of medical knowledge and find ways to integrate this information into the workflows of their increasingly busy and chaotic lives in the clinic. This is no easy task. Later in this book, we will take a look at the field of big data and the computing tools that are making it possible to scan millions of pages of medical literature and integrate this knowledge and data with the observations of the clinician to improve clinician's decision-making. Integration of data analytics with wireless technologies will become increasingly common over the coming years. We also have new tools that both clinician and patient can use together to make more informed decisions when multiple therapeutic options are available. These types of tools can both improve outcomes and save money. As more patients utilize wireless tracking devices to monitor their conditions and remote monitoring becomes more ubiquitous, we run the risk of drowning in a sea of data. This is where the role of technologies such as big data and data analytics will become invaluable to manage vast amount of streaming data and to make sense of all of these data. Just collecting data for data's sake does not solve many problems. Fortunately, there are many entrepreneurs and companies working at the nexus of wireless health and data to help the system and individuals manage these pain points. What lies on the horizon is an important shift in medicine. Historically, medicine has been based on retrospective studies and data and episodic encounters with patients. With anytime/anyplace health that wireless devices create, *we are beginning to see the rise of real-time, real-world medicine* based on many data points beyond a single medical encounter. Here, we will see innovations that not only improve the quality of care, but also offer substantial savings and efficiencies across the health system.

The estimated cost of reforming the healthcare system to cover all Americans is $1 trillion over 10 years, as healthcare futurist Joe Flower observes.[16] He highlights this fact to remind us that inefficiencies and waste account for over $750–780 billion per year which is nearly *eight times what it would cost to insure all currently uninsured Americans.* Healthcare waste exceeds the 2009 budget for the department of defense. Of the estimated $600 million spent on laboratory tests, approximately 70 % of these funds are spent on paperwork. Flower's insights should bring home the realization of what is possible if we can put into place the mechanisms for creating a rationally organized and managed healthcare system. If we can transition to a prevention economy that can bring down the rates of chronic diseases through wireless technologies combined with more effective behavioral change modalities, decrease medical errors through checklists and sensors, improve physician workflows with well-designed EHRs and clinical decision support, and coordinate care more effectively through the cloud—a lot of "IFS"—but perfectly feasible within a decade. Below, we provide a brief overview of the sources of excess costs in the system identified by the Institute of Medicine in 2010. Many of these are areas where appropriate technologies combined with business practices and incentives could result in tremendous savings:

- Utilization of unnecessary services ($210 billion)

  - Overuse, beyond evidence-based standards
  - Unnecessary use of higher cost services

- Inefficiently delivered services ($130 billion)

  - Mistakes, errors
  - Fragmented care
  - Unnecessary use of higher cost providers
  - Operational inefficiencies

- Excess administrative costs ($190 billion)

  - Insurance paperwork costs beyond benchmarks
  - Insurers' administrative inefficiencies
  - Inefficiencies due to care documentation requirements

- Price inefficiencies ($105 billion)
  - Products and services not in alignment with benchmarks
- Lack of prevention services and savings ($55 billion)
- Fraud ($75 billion)

One of the perplexing issues with health care is how irrational it appears to the laymen. Trust us, when you devote your professional career to health and medicine, this perception does not go away because the economics of health care rarely fit within prevailing economic paradigms, nor does it resemble anything remotely

---

[16]Joe Flower (2012). Healthcare Beyond Reform. Doing it Right for Half the Cost.

rational as the diabetes case discussed earlier illustrates. An analogy often used to get the point across is to imagine if grocery stores were like health care. You would buy your groceries, and after passing through the checkout, you would have no idea what your groceries cost because you would not get a bill for another month or so. Drug prices across hospitals and plans can vary by an order of magnitude or more. There is a great deal of talk about "consumer-driven" health care that assumes that there is a market in health care that resembles some kind of mythical rational market where information on prices is perfectly transparent. The challenge often goes beyond information asymmetries to just plain dysfunctional markets. Joe Flower makes the case clearly when he observes that there are useful treatments for back pain that may cost several hundred dollars and they compete unsuccessfully against alternatives for \$50,000–75,000.[17] In later chapters, we will explore some of the platforms that belong to the Health 2.0 space that are targeting the lack of **transparency** to create more consumer-friendly platforms that enable patients to obtain an accurate estimate of what actual costs will be for a given procedure as well as which providers have the best record of good outcomes for that procedure. One can see through examples such as the XeoHealth and MediKredit Integrated Health Consulting collaboration to automate the adjudication of claims that digital technologies can both cut administrative waste and improve the experience for patients dealing with both health insurance companies and their providers. Dealing with both of these parties is a source of immense frustration for patients caught in the middle. This process is known as "real-time adjudication" of claims, and it is already a reality in South Africa, but feels like a distant dream still in the USA for most consumers outside of the contexts where XeoHealth is deployed.

Wireless Health and the Health IT Ecosystem: The Technology that Is Driving Change

The technologies that are creating the possibilities for health system transformation include mobiles, cloud computing, social networks, data analytics platforms, telehealth, and sensors. Most of these technologies are familiar and have become globalized technologies over the past decade. In fact, in some ways, the USA was behind in adoption of mobile phones for health care compared to some countries in Africa and Asia where the "mHealth revolution" has been underway for nearly a decade. In contexts where health professionals are in short supply, the mobile phone has become a necessary technology for extending the reach of the health-care system into villages. From Bangladesh to South Africa and beyond, we have seen very innovative uses of mobile phones to remind women of when to have checkups for their antenatal care when pregnant, to remind HIV sufferers to take

---

[17]Ibid, p. 44.

their life-saving antiretroviral medications, or to collect data on health issues that inform how health systems will allocate resources. It has come as a surprise at times when we spoke to US audiences several years ago about mHealth, and the first question out of the lips of public health academics was that how will the poor use new technologies because they lack access. All we need to do is look at the numbers. Cell phones are ubiquitous in much of the developing world and the USA. Sure, we can find pockets where poverty rates are extremely high and they are not found in 100 % of the population. Smartphones are steadily making inroads globally as well. Even in the USA, we find that nearly 50 % of the population has a smartphone. In the coming years, as Moore's law brings down the price of smartphones, we even expect to find them in very large numbers in places like Kenya. Do not be surprised if in the next few years you come across companies providing mHealth applications and services that originated in Kenya, South Africa, or India.

To give you an idea of just how ubiquitous the cell phone is—probably the most successful technology ever created—we will look at some of the global and US data and you will easily see why the mobile platform is one of the most promising ways to get health information, and care, into the hands of the most people. At the end of last year, according to the International Telecommunications Union, there were nearly 6 billion cell phone subscriptions.[18] This is not the same as saying 6 billion people out of a total global population of 7 billion have access to mobiles due to the fact that many people have more than one.

The Pew Foundation regularly researches the role of mobiles and information and communication technologies in American life. These surveys are useful in creating a reality check of the distribution and use of various devices and their potential for health applications. What is striking is the decline of landlines and how mobiles are increasingly displacing the use of traditional landlines. Cell phone access greatly exceeds other computing platforms in terms of access as the numbers below indicate. In 2015, the Pew Research Center found that 2/3 of Americans are now using smartphones and 10 % of Americans own a smartphone but do not have access to broadband. For many low-income households, the smartphone is the primary source of health information. For the elderly, smartphone use is growing, but we still have a way to go to leverage these tools to improve outcomes in a scalable way with elderly populations. We will examine this challenge later when we dive deeper into the future of aging technologies and we will see a number of creative solutions that attempt to work around this challenge and design products specifically for the needs of the elderly.

Today's smartphones are far more than a phone. Your camera can be used to measure your heart rate. Peripheral devices such as microscopes and diagnostics can turn the phone into a small laboratory to diagnose malaria. An additional sensor, such as the device developed by AliveCor, can enable it to do an ECG, and a company that the author is involved with, Ram Group, will soon have the next

---

[18]http://www.itu.int/ITU-D/ict/facts/2011/material/ICTFactsFigures2011.pdf.

generation of hemodynamic sensors that do far more at an even lower price point. The accelerometer can detect a fall, and sensors in the shoes can detect changes in gait that are predictive of the onset of dementia. Apps have plenty of data to help you do everything from finding a doctor or scheduling an appointment (ZocDoc) to planning your diet. The Withings body scale and blood pressure cuff can track and record your weight and blood pressure on an app on your phone or iPad so that the next time you are in the doctor's office you have many data points rather than a single point to draw upon in his or her diagnostic process. The Apple iTunes store now has over 60,000 apps under health and medicine. The problem is that most are not based on any sound science whatsoever, and only 1 in 50 is connected to a health professional. There is a plenty of room in the marketplace for curators of apps who can help both clinicians and patients wade through the thicket of apps to find those that are based on best practices and science and offer consumers the knowledge to make the right choices on digital health offerings.

Sensors are another important technology in today's health technology ecosystem. From RFID tags to sensors that measure temperature, pollutant levels, respiration, location, and countless other indicators, we are beginning to enter a world where the number of phenomena that are being monitored by sensors is exploding. Many of these sensors are connected to the Internet to form what is called "the Internet of Things." In reality, we have a Health Internet of Things when we take into account the remote monitoring technologies, and sensors monitoring health and environmental conditions are assembled together. During the aftermath of the 2011 Japanese tsunami and the nuclear reactor crisis in Fukushima, there was an interesting use of sensors for broader public health concerns that is illustrative. An open source sensor technology developed by Pachube (now renamed as Cosm, then Xively) was deployed by citizens throughout Japan and the Asia-Pacific region to monitor radiation levels. These sensors could transmit data to the Internet, and radiation levels could be monitored by anyone with access to the site. Trust in the Japanese government's public statements on radiation levels was undermined when citizen sensor networks indicated much higher levels than the government would admit. Similar types of sensors are in use in a number of environmental health contexts from China to the UK. These examples illustrate one of the powerful lessons of these new technologies in health—that is, there is a great potential to democratize data collection and public debate over expertise in these matters. No longer will data and the interpretation of data be left in the hands of a small elite. Citizen science is coming and becoming more and more powerful every day. Technologies are embedded in networks of meaning and political action and not just matters for health IT experts to discuss with themselves in digital health conferences.

The number of things connected to the Internet is growing dramatically: Estimates range from 20 billion[19] to 50 billion[20] connected devices by 2020. In

---

[19]IMS Research, "Internet Connected Devices About to Pass the 5 Billion Milestone," August 19, 2010, press release.

[20]Djuphammar, Hakan, Ericsson, in Lamberth (p. 9).

2008, the number of things connected to the Internet exceeded the number of people on Earth for the first time.[21] A growing number of these devices are linked to the health sector and may offer new insights into the connections between the body and the environment. Later we will learn how sensors that stream data in real time from remote monitoring devices in the home or in clinical settings can be linked to sophisticated data analytics platforms and lead to important new clinical insights that had been overlooked by clinicians and researchers. The challenge here is the issue of data deluge and having the computing power to make sense of all of the data.

Health 2.0: Social Networks and Health

The growth and scale of social networks such as Twitter and Facebook have made even many of the naysayers who were skeptics about social media stand up and take note of the potential that social networking platforms can play in health care. We are now seeing a number of successful platforms that connect patients and/or physicians. Some interesting examples that have taken off in recent years include the closed network for physicians, Sermo, that enables physicians to share and exchange clinical insights. The community currently has over 125,000 physicians from 68 specialties with a number of research collaborations through academic research centers. Online communities such as Sermo provide an important forum for clinicians to dialog about innovative strategies, best practices, and research. In this book, we have the founder of **Tabeeb**, a new Medicine 2.0 site that focuses on crowd-sourcing medical insights for difficult-to-solve cases, discuss how social businesses can use cooperation more effectively to create both successful businesses, and solve serious social challenges linked to access to medical care and knowledge.

From the patient perspective, Health 2.0 networks have offered a myriad of communities for patients to find other patients for mutual support and sharing of experiences. Many of these platforms are growing in sophistication as the ability to collect and share data from personal health records (PHRs), tracking devices, and members of the so-called quantified self (people who track activity levels, diet, health outcomes, and often experiment with new lifestyle regimens). The well-known site, PatientsLikeMe.com, has become a beacon for the potential of Health 2.0 sites to build a community of patients and contribute to treatments of diseases. PatientsLikeMe was founded by the brother of a patient who died from Lou Gehrig's disease or ALS. After witnessing his brother's struggle, Jamie Heywood created the site for ALS sufferers to share their experiences. This rapidly evolved into a platform where patients could track the progress of their disease and use of medications. As more patients began to participate, an interesting thing

---

[21]http://blogs.cisco.com/news/the-Internet-of-things-infographic/.

happened. Most physicians will have only had experience treating a small number of ALS sufferers; therefore, they do not have a large number of cases to draw upon to inform optimization of therapies. But when a large number of ALS patients chart their own outcomes as a community, this can provide an amazing resource for physicians to understand individual responses to specific drugs through larger sample sizes beyond their own practice. Eventually, this community of patients entered the fray of what now goes by a number of names including "citizen science," "participatory science," and "expert patient-led science" and published some of the first peer-reviewed medical journal articles based on their own findings about commonly used treatments for ALS. Health 2.0 is changing how new scientific knowledge is produced.

PatientsLikeMe is only one of many communities that are now available. Alliance Health Networks, MedHelp, TuDiabetes, Daily Strength, CureTogether, the list could go on for quite a bit. The many-to-many Web or Web 2.0 platforms have created the means for patients, particularly those with rare disorders, to find "communities of practice," so to speak, where they can link to motivate one another, share their experiences, launch campaigns for cures, and participate in collective research efforts. Some of these platforms have begun to scale reaching over 100,000 individuals in several cases. PatientsLikeMe currently has over 125,000 users and extends well beyond ALS to nearly 500 different diseases or conditions. A personal genomics platform (an early start-up) for crowd-sourcing genetics research, GenomEra, has well over 300 individuals sharing personal genetic data for research efforts. What is interesting about these networks is who is doing the science—patients and laypersons. Open innovation has come to the health and medical sciences in some very important ways. The tools of scientific research, data, and platforms are democratizing who can do what. Even in relatively new technology areas such as big data, there are open source and inexpensive ways for laypersons with training from open courseware or Massive Online Open Courseware (MOOC) such as Coursera and Big Data University (IBM's online training platform for their big data tools) to analyze large datasets or conduct data mining on Twitter and other social networking platforms.

One of the technologies that are enabling mobiles, social networks, and big data to drive structural changes in health care is the cloud. **Cloud computing** is essentially the use of hardware such as servers and software to deliver computing services over the Internet.[22] Rather than installing software on your computer, a method that is increasingly viewed as "old-fashioned," you log into a Web site and can utilize the software online. This is referred to as software-as-a-service, but one can find a number of different types of cloud services including platform-as-a-service, data-as-a-service, and API-as-a-service, and recently, Microsoft and IBM began offering Blockchain-as-a-service. The significance of the cloud is that it offers the opportunity to scale computing power and share services more readily. This is why the cloud is critically important to health care. In our discussion on

---

[22]https://en.wikipedia.org/wiki/Cloud_computing.

inefficiencies, we noted the fragmentation in the healthcare system that most often leads to data locked in silos where it remains unused or difficult to access. Why spend money collecting data if we do not use it to improve the quality of care? For too long, security of data trumped ease of use and access by the right people. This is beginning to change, and we are beginning to see a great deal of innovation at the nexus of data and the cloud that will enable us to do things in the healthcare system that were quite challenging before. Security and privacy will remain important concerns, but no longer can we hide behind the firewalls of security and leave the quality of care to suffer. Over the next few years, as healthcare providers are incentivized to coordinate care and are paid for performance rather than strictly by a fee-for-service reimbursement mechanism, the cloud combined with powerful data analytics will be crucial to the economic and medical success of medical practice. Cloud computing provides the connective tissue to share patient data and manage care remotely and a platform for analyzing the data. Consumer-facing tools in the mHealth space are also reliant on cloud computing via their apps. Data stored in the cloud will be the glue that ties healthcare providers and patients working together to improve health and well-being.

The Algorithmic Revolution in Health care

The political economist John Zysman from the University of California at Berkeley has been studying various "digital revolutions" over the past two decades and the growing role for algorithms in various parts of the economy. Many services in the economy are gradually being transformed into codifiable and comput-able processes and implemented by IT tools.[23] Algorithmic revolutions are accompanied by service revolutions, and these are not the services of "service economies" past that are low-wage, low-value-added nature. These are the new engines of economic productivity and offer the opportunity to transform entire sectors of the economy into new business models, new ways to organize the firm, new skills and knowledge assets, and even new classes of professionals. Algorithms are automating many tasks, including many of the processes involved in health care. This book is essentially the story of the algorithmic revolution in health care and how it will transform the way we think about health care, how it is provided, and where value will be created in the future.

The algorithmic and service revolutions typically blur the boundary between the product and the service. Think about Apple and the introduction of the iPod in the early 2000s. The innovation really was not just about the iPod but the com-bination of the iPod and iTunes together. In one swoop, Steve Jobs and his col-leagues at Apple figured out how to get your credit card number in exchange for access to entertainment on their product. This was a very different business

---

[23]http://brie.berkeley.edu/publications/wp171.pdf.

model and service from what came before and had a dramatic effect on how we experience music. The App Store has had a similar effect. The iPhone once again introduced the concept of the App Store and an entire eco-system of apps otherwise known as the App Economy. A few short years since the introduction of the iPhone 3, we have largely forgotten how this innovation fundamentally reshaped the market for cell phones. Android has had a similar effect, but in the open source arena that increasingly competes with Apple. Platforms connect producers of content with the consumers of content and have fundamentally transformed the economy if we think about Google, Amazon, Facebook, and Apple. Why hasn't this happened in health care yet and what kind of platform could transform the current non-system into one that better serves the needs of patients and providers? We hear much talk about the Uber of health care, but I am guessing we need to search for a different model that takes health equity and fairness into consideration. Health is a public good and just calling it "consumer-driven" so we can take more out of patients' pockets will not work either.

Health care is in the early days of a similar technological revolution, but the trajectory will likely be very different. The closed system of Apple resembles the legacy systems of eHealth technologies that are part of the problem that many new start-ups in wireless health services are attempting to disrupt. Apple is beginning to do some interesting work in digital health with the introduction of apps such as ResearchKit, HealthKit, and CareKit. However, an open eco-system that has a similar effect of enabling consumer-friendly generation of data, *sharing of data*, integration of data, and analytical capabilities that create actionable insights could be a major game changer and is more relevant to health care than the proprietary model that Apple espouses. The platform wars for digital health have already begun as by mid-2014 Google, Apple, Samsung, WebMD, and Microsoft have all announced major initiatives with the first three being the most aggressive in the race to become the central system integrator for health and/or wellness data. In a sense, we are living in the version 1.0 Era of the algorithmic revolution where we have lots of devices collecting data. But no single player has quite yet become the "health layer" to integrate all of these data, make sense of it, and offer the data-as-a-service in a manner that is the game changer for patients, clinicians, and the health system in general. One can see elements of this in the current ecosystem where service providers like RunKeeper enable users to track and share data from their workouts, but also integrate data from various fitness devices and trackers such as Withings scales and blood pressure cuffs. Qualcomm has developed the 2Net hub to integrate Wifi- and Bluetooth-enabled health devices in the home via a simple-to-use plug-and-play device. We will likely see new entrants into the healthcare marketplace often from unexpected quarters. That smart TV that you have read about in Wired Magazine can become a portal for the delivery of health content in the medical home (although we need to first figure out what to do about inadvertent messaging about one's Viagra prescription during your Thanksgiving football viewing with family and friends!). Those medical devices previously used in the hospital might become much more desirable devices when the Apple's and other consumer electronics companies decide to redesign them for the mass market.

But beyond the devices and gadgets, it will be important to not lose sight of the key challenges and opportunities that the algorithmic revolution in health care will touch. Opportunities for more personalized therapies and lifestyle coaching based on one's multiple streams of health data—genomic, lifestyle, fitness, biomarkers, prescription history, environmental context, and social network analytics (strength of social ties, social cohesiveness of neighborhoods, walkability, and built environment)—all can be influenced by feedback loops that the combination of data and technology will empower. For example, at UCLA, the Personal Environmental Impact Report platform utilizes sensors to track your movements and environmental context to provide insights on pollutants that may trigger your asthma based on geolocation but **also tracks your** contribution to environmental pollutant levels based on your driving behavior.[24] TicTrac is another service that facilitates aggregation of tracking data, but still, the data feedback services have a way to go before becoming a truly robust data service. The missing component of the current generation of wearables is the personalized coaching that makes sense of data beyond pretty data visualizations and offers feedback to the user. We are beginning to see algorithm-driven services such as these through coaching engines and services offered by Performance Lab (New Zealand) and Omada Health in the USA. We still have a long way to go, however.

What is emerging is a new paradigm of personalized medicine or Personalized Medicine 2.0. The first generation of thinking in this area was fueled by the biotech revolution from the late 1980s into the early 2000s up to the mapping of the human genome. In 2003, systems biologist Lee Hood coined the term "4P Medicine" where the 4Ps were the following:

- Predictive
- Personalized
- Preventive
- Participatory

His vision was informed by biology, but he recognized early on the need for more robust IT systems in medical research and health care. The vision is one where genetics can provide early detection of illness based on one's individual genome and then take action to prevent the onset of illness for many diseases that have a lifestyle or curative dimension available. This would require the active engagement of the patient. Since he originally developed the concept of 4P Medicine, much has changed on the IT front, however. The participatory nature of the social Web or Web 2.0 plus the integration of data points from outside the body such as environmental data, social network analysis, and the mobile platform has grown such that 4P Medicine can have an even more systemic or integrative vision that

---

[24]http://www.eecs.ucf.edu/~turgut/COURSES/EEL6788_AWN_Spr11/Papers/Mun-PersonalEnvironmentalImpactReport.pdf.

ties together genomics, environmental health, and the so-called socialization of illness (i.e., the role that social determinants and social networks and supports have in both the spread of chronic diseases and role in disease management). For the biologists out there, we have a more expansive possibility with wireless health to integrate the genome with the other systems: metabolome, microbiome,[25] enviromentome, connectome,[26] and diseaseome.[27] This is a long-term process but where we are most certainly headed in the coming decades. In other words, personalized medicine needs to have a much stronger digital services role that can integrate these other data streams from the environment, behavior, and social context with one's genomic and medical data, so true personalization can happen while also enabling population-based health approaches to grow as well. The new era of value-based care is making population-based approaches more valuable and they could be made much more cost-effective and therapeutic with better data analytics built upon diverse data streams. Personalized medicine and population health management do not necessarily have to be at odds with one another. Some ethicists are concerned about the focus on personalized medicine that may exclude population-based approaches, but we believe that the cooperative approaches espoused in this book can offer bridges between the two and ease this tension. True platform strategies, if designed with the right incentives, could drive innovation across these two poles as well.

The insights from both the sciences and how our social interactions are increasingly mediated through the Web are offering up a very different paradigm for health. If we bring together the notion of more expansive personal health ecologies or resources that people now draw upon to manage and understand their health and well-being; open innovation that has opened up the walls of the laboratory and company to novel sources of knowledge and innovation; and the vast eco-system of digital or wireless health technologies, we are actually entering into a new world of "Open Health." One interesting data point to consider here is the example of Foldit, an online game developed by researchers at the University of Washington in 2011, which was developed to solve a scientific problem that professional researchers had failed to solve for more than a decade. The challenge was to understand the three-dimensional structure of enzymes important for the development of novel therapeutics for HIV. Foldit was developed as an online game where laypersons could rapidly learn how to manipulate 3D models of proteins online. Large numbers of online participants played the online game and essentially solved puzzles by manipulating the proteins by following the simple

---

[25]For a general overview of the microbiome written for the non-specialist, see Michael Specter's "Germs Are Us" in the New Yorker: http://www.newyorker.com/reporting/2012/10/22/121022fa_fact_specter.

[26]http://www.ted.com/talks/sebastian_seung.html.

[27]Melanie Swan, 2012. J. Pers. Med. Health 2050: The Realization of Personalized Medicine through Crowdsourcing, the Quantified Self, and the Participatory Biocitizen. 2, 93–118; doi: 10.3390/jpm20300093.

game mechanics built around the physics of the atomic structures. They helped build insights on the "recipes" for protein structures by playing the game which in turn helped build algorithms that were more effective than the most commonly used bioinformatics software. They pulled this off in weeks without formally understanding exactly what they were doing.[28] Game players illustrated how very complex solutions could be discovered at a fraction of the cost of conventional science if they only had the proper environment and systems to collaborate. This illustrates the power of co-creation and crowd-sourcing to solve medical problems. We explore this later in the book in our chapter by Osama Alshaykh.

Engaged patients using sophisticated tracking tools; peer-to-peer platforms for sharing ideas, data, and knowledge; gamification in both wellness and research; tools for generating greater transparency in health care and medicine; new data commons; and crowd-sourcing and crowd-funding models—these all intersect with the innovations in wireless health in transformative ways. In the mid-1990s, anthropologist Paul Rabinow wrote a seminal essay on new forms of sociality that were arising out of the growth of biological knowledge.[29] He termed this change *biosociality* to explain how people are connecting and identifying themselves increasingly on the basis of biological knowledge such as one's disease status. The trends and developments we are documenting in this book are the next stage of biosociality—when it becomes digital or digital biosociality and how this will shape health care in the future. This is a world with greater participation by patients themselves in research and setting up the research agenda for collecting the data. Biosociality will also demand new thinking on ethics and politics as well. The ethics of algorithms and where and which humans intervene to avoid discrimination, gender bias, and racisms that can be embodied in the categories used for data and data collection will need much more consideration.

While we often focus on the health policy agendas that are set from above, what is important here is how more bottom-up engagement is accelerating, thanks to the democratization of knowledge. Influential "ePatients" have become spokespersons for what they view as wrong with the current health system and are actively involved in developing the technologies, policies, and social communities that will shape the future. This will no doubt be viewed as threatening in some quarters used to the maxim that "doctor or scientist knows best." Other physicians and scientists will recognize the opportunities, as well as the dangers, and figure out ways to harness this energy to improve the quality of care and the development of new therapies and even address the financial dilemmas that our healthcare system raises. We increasingly hear critiques of smart cities initiatives as too technocentric and top-down and in need of greater citizen engagement. But citizen engagement is not easy and will never be the cure-all for these initiatives, but we

[28]http://blogs.discovermagazine.com/notrocketscience/2011/11/07/computer-gamers-foldit-protein-algorithm/.

[29]Rabinow, P. (1996) "Artificiality and enlightenment: from sociobiology to biosociality" in *Essays on the Anthropology of Reason*. Princeton: Princeton University Press.

must still work on solutions that begin small and can scale in ethically appropriate ways. Cooperation is often messy, hard to manage, yet necessary. As we travel in this new landscape, we will need to develop the analytical tools to sort the hype and hope from the realities. Our health system is not an easy beast to tame. In fact, many start-ups have been eaten alive by the fragmentation and perverse incentives. We cannot always believe the breathless hype of technology blogs promising new revolutions in a single platform or new technology. It is a system after all, but we have decided to write this book at the current conjecture because we truly do believe it is an important tipping point for medicine and health care. More than ever, we need strategic and innovative forms of cooperation to actually deliver the promise of better care in an affordable manner. This is something both sides of the political aisle and stakeholders across the political spectrum can find common cause in fixing a broken system. Earlier in this chapter, we mentioned how most healthcare challenges are examples of "wicked problems" where no single approach will solve the problem. There may never be a drug to cure obesity, stress, or the health consequences of poverty. Therefore, having the leadership skills and creativity to drive innovation that entails moving complex value chains and systems (even eco-systems) of stakeholders to align their business models and strategies may require skills that few of us have learned in the university or even in the firms where we work. We want to show in the chapters that follow that we do not need to reinvent the wheel when it comes to cooperation, but rather we may need to change mind-sets about who and how health care is delivered, what we value in health and well-being, and how we work, as societies to produce better health outcomes. What this points to is the innovation in *meaning* that will need to accompany the devices and business models that transform health systems in the future.

So what is disruptive cooperation? Helga Nowotny[30] in her meditation on innovation notes the distinction between "the new" and innovation. She makes the observation that in European–American sign language, the sign for the future points forward, but in African sign language, it points to the rear. We see the future through what appears in the past and present. We cannot start from scratch with health system transformation and have to work with the structures that are present. Our "workarounds" are working around what we have already created. But digital health and design, when done right, should aim to design for desired health outcomes rather than purely on existing healthcare infrastructures. This approach will undoubtedly be dismissed by those who see the legacy technology players in health care and the electronic health record providers, for example, as an unshakable cartel. But we beg to differ. We see the seeds of cooperation in the growing use of crowd-sourcing, open innovation, DIY health, and new ways of thinking about the Internet that Blockchain, as one example, provides, as opening up new opportunities. Transforming systems will require a myriad of actors, public–private partnerships, business model transformations to move from fee-for-service to value-based care, and a world of population health management. Managing

---

[30]Helga Nowotny. 2008. Insatiable Curiosity. Innovation in a Fragile Future. MIT Press.

complex partnerships and eco-systems requires leadership capable of communicating solutions across eco-systems with widely different worldviews and opinions on the problem, as well as an ability to revisit assumptions about how health care operates, a difficult thing to accomplish as the Obama Administration has learned. Nevertheless, there are tools and approaches coming from outside of health care that could provide a platform to build complex solutions and platforms that can make the challenge easier to surmount than we often think *within health care.* Nowotny thinks *we need to oscillate between seriousness and play, science, and irony, and we would add competition and cooperation, the market, and public goods, to build a better future for health care.* Innovation in health care cannot be just a new fashion trend for new apps and devices alone. If we took existing products off the shelves and optimized use of them within well-functioning systems, we could easily hit the triple aim of quality care, access to care at a lower cost. Unfortunately, a legacy of perverse incentives, structural dysfunction, antiquated business models, and the world beyond health systems makes this far more difficult than it should be. The leadership to manage complex forms of cooperation is urgently needed, and we hope this volume can provide at least a few tools to help others think in new ways. We cannot escape the systems of the past, nor do we have to be completely bound by their constraints. We hope this book is a start for building new conversations across the divides and disciplines that often keep us from thinking about health systems and can contribute to building more patient-friendly, real-world, resilient, and accountable health systems in the future.

I will end this introduction with a brief parable and autobiographical note about political change. In 1989, I was a graduate student in Bologna, Italy, and in January of that year, I visited Prague, Czechoslovakia, and befriended a young journalism student. In July 1989, I returned to spend a week with my new found friend. On each end of that week, I had the opportunity to witness the fall of communism in Hungary and Poland as political forces came together to dismantle the communist regimes. On the way from Hungary to Poland with a stop in Prague, I smuggled a copy of Newsweek that had an interview with the former National Security Advisor to President Jimmy Carter, Zbigniew Brzezinski. Professor Brzezinski, with whom I took a class with merely two months later, was quoted for predicting that the Czech regime would fall within two years. I showed the article to my Czech friend who scoffed, "It will take twice as long as that, the regime is in firm control." Fortunately, several months later, I received a letter in the mail with a flyer that was used to call the citizenry to the streets and protest the brutal behavior of the regime. The Velvet Revolution had overturned the regime with little bloodshed. No one predicted this. The pervasive feeling one has working on health care often leaves one feeling that poorly designed technology is our destiny. But poorly designed technology is not safe for patients, drives up the cost of care, and leads to negative experiences of health care and wellness for the entire population. We can do better, and accepting the status quo is no longer acceptable. As healthcare professionals and citizens, it is time that we think beyond the hubris of "there is an app for that" on the one hand and tolerating the status quo on the other. In 2015, the former head of the National Office for the Coordination of Health Information Technology (ONC) made a call for a "day of action" where one million patients would demand that provider systems provide access to their health data. The fact that this cry even needs to be made is, well, ridiculous and illustrates the lack of leadership in health technology. It is embarrassing. If health care is going to become truly patient-centric, it just cannot be left to headers on PowerPoint decks at health IT conferences and we need to develop the tools that actually engage citizens in healthcare technology design and the co-creation of health outcomes in a manner that is equitable and not just cost-shifting. This would be disruptive cooperation.

Chapter 2
Patients, Platforms, and Wearables: Co-creating Value from Health Data and Wearables

Jody Ranck

In 2002, Venezuelan-born Manny Hernandez received his first diagnosis of diabetes. Living in Arizona at the time, he was 30, overweight, and told he had type II diabetes. Over the next several months he struggled to keep control over his condition and by early 2003 his family doctor ran out of ideas, and the traditional therapies were not working, so he was referred to an endocrinologist. The endocrinologist tested his HbA1c (hemoglobin A1c is an important indicator that measures how well one's diabetes is being controlled) and antibody levels and realized that Manny actually had type I diabetes and immediately prescribed an insulin regime that included long-acting insulin as well as watching his carbohydrate intake levels. In 2005, he received an insulin pump that helped to make his diabetes more manageable. The difference an insulin pump makes for a diabetic is rather dramatic. Rather than requiring 20-30 shots of insulin over 3 days he only required one shot from the pump.

Manny's experience with diabetes for the first several years was rather typical. Typical in the sense that he did not know anyone else with his condition. But this changed in 2006 when he participated in a diabetes patient group in Orlando, Florida, and for the first time met many people like himself. This experience planted a seed for an idea—he and his wife decided to try to replicate this experience and created a new platform for diabetics. TuDiabetes.org was created in March 2007 and a Spanish version, Estudiabetes.org was launched in August 2007. This would become a major online meeting place for diabetics to share their experiences with the disease and insights on how to manage it. Social supports have been well known in public health as important aspects of health outcomes and platforms such as TuDiabetes were becoming a growing force in healthcare

J. Ranck (✉)
Health Bank, Ranck Consulting, Ram Group, Washington, DC, USA
e-mail: jody@ranckconsulting.com

© Springer International Publishing Switzerland 2016

29

J. Ranck (ed.), *Disruptive Cooperation in Digital Health*,
DOI 10.1007/978-3-319-40980-1_2

early on in the so-called Web 2.0 revolution. Their first online campaign was the "Palm of your hand" campaign that asked people to write how they feel about life with diabetes on the palm of their hands. They collected approximately 100 or so "hands" and created a video about their experiences. This campaign caught the attention of LifeScan, a company that makes devices for diabetics, who made a donation that helped Manny to launch the Diabetes Hands Foundation by March 2008.

Since these early days TuDiabetes has developed into one of the most active diabetes patient platforms. TuDiabetes was created on the social networking platform Ning and they have developed a Ning app, TuAnalyze (developed in collaboration with the Centers for Disease Control and Prevention), that has a personal health record (PHR) connected that allows patients to collect their self-care data (A1c levels) that they track and share it with whomever they want. This has become useful in some of the campaigns that TuDiabetes runs such as the Big Blue test that encourages diabetics to exercise and test their blood glucose levels. Diabetics from around the world have participated in the campaign and they also have the ability to share videos documenting their experiences. TuDiabetes, through the TuAnalyze application, also contributes to research through collaboration with the Children's Hospital of Boston where they have analyzed the data that participants shared. There is a gap in the public health research on diabetes where a lack of understanding of people's locations and testing behaviors or the impact of social networks on diabetes care. The TuAnalyze platform also makes it easy to create surveys that can be used for additional research. To date the research has shown that engagement with social networks over time can significantly improve consistent testing of A1c levels which in turn leads to better health outcomes.

One of the impacts of this type of online community is to amplify the power of patient voices in major policy decisions whether at the FDA or in insurance plans. They now have a platform to aggregate their voices and exert their pressure on health insurers to purchase technologies that are best for the patient rather than make decisions based on the cheapest product. In the past, many diabetics in the TuDiabetes community have viewed purchasing decisions by some health plans as more in the interest of the plan than the patient. They are now becoming experts in navigating a complex health system and advocate for the technology options that serve their needs best. Later we discuss the People Powered Health approach fostered by NESTA in the UK that focuses on building on the knowledge and capabilities of patient groups and communities. We need to think about how new technologies and business models can engage with these practices as part of what we call "innovation."

Enabling Patient and Researcher Collaborations

The story of TuDiabetes and the collaboration with clinical researchers is a signal of a growing part of the way in which digital health is changing the traditional relationships in research and the practice of medicine. There are numerous efforts underway to augment the role of patients in clinical trials and research efforts through more participatory approaches. Online patient communities have offered new platforms for engaging with patients in the aggregate that can be quite valuable to research efforts. In order to continue to build on these efforts, there are a number of technological and policy issues that can be improved upon to make it easier to connect patients and researchers. It is estimated that only 4 % of Americans are aware of a clinical trial that they could potentially participate in and help further the growth of medical knowledge. Apple's ResearchKit application launched in early 2015 illustrates how new tools and platforms can fundamentally alter the way we design trials when in the first 36 h of its existence the ResearchKit app enabled more new participants in clinical research efforts than would normally have been enrolled if 50 medical centers spent a year in recruiting participants.

One of the missing elements has been a viable way for the consumer or citizen to store the data that are collected from their devices and then have a relatively simple way of exchanging the data with researchers or clinicians in a private and secure manner. Google's early efforts in health via GoogleHealth was an early venture to create a Personal Health Record (PHR) that could store patient-generated data and also have links to research institutions and health providers. The problem was that there was not enough patient-generated data available and the underlying business case was not robust in the mid-2000s to support growth in use of the PHR. Microsoft Vault has been slightly more successful and has enabled integration with a wide range of tracking devices and platforms as well as ways to integrate your prescription data from your pharmacy and other health-related services. There is still a problem of not having a robust enough use case to really create a business providing a "must-have" service to consumers. This has led many observers of digital health to conclude that the PHR is simply not going to work in the current digital health ecosystem. Or, can we rethink the PHR from a passive storage receptacle to become something akin to a patient platform where patients can do things with data and transactions can take place?

This is the novel approach that a Swiss start-up that the author of this chapter is involved with has taken. Healthbank, a Swiss-based start-up, has built a platform that is designed to offer a secure, private storage service for consumer health data but incentivize data sharing and harvesting greater public good from moving data out of silos. Most surveys show that citizens of Europe and the USA are very interested in sharing health data in a private and secure way if medical research and public health can benefit.

The User Experience   ✚ healthbank

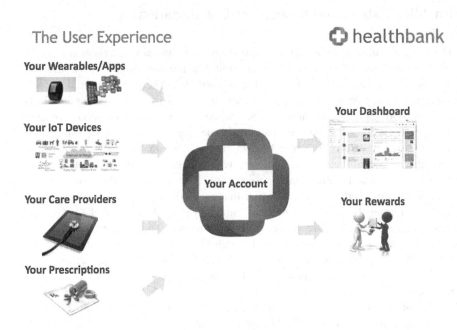

Your Wearables/Apps

Your IoT Devices

Your Care Providers

Your Prescriptions

Your Dashboard

Your Account

Your Rewards

Healthbank is a cooperative business model where citizens who become members also are co-owners and have a voting role in corporate governance. In a world where consumers are increasingly concerned with the manner in which companies use their data in unauthorized ways, we feel that a cooperative model can help build trust and become part of a system that incentivizes doing more with data and putting the patient or citizen in control of who gets to use their data.

So why is this important now? Cardiologist Eric Topol and Leonard Kish spell this out in a paper in Nature, "Unpatients—Why patients should own their own medical data"[1] The authors point out the dramatically lower cost in sequencing whole-genome data and the growth in biological and medical data that is skyrocketing every year. And this is not just the volume of data or big data, but data over the entire life history of individuals leading to "long data" or a longitudinal record of a person that can be analyzed over the life course for predictive or personalized medicine types of care. The problem is that there is no centralized place to bring together EHR data, patient-generated data, and genetic data and this is a problem for actually implementing precision medicine initiatives. We also need to not lose sight of population health approaches as we increasingly personalize care. In most of the USA, the existing legal frameworks empower physicians and hospitals to own the patient's data. The authors argue that in no other sector of the economy do we see consumers responsible for paying for a good but someone else owns the good afterward. But this is the reality of your health data. The legal status of

---

[1]Leonard Kish and Eric Topol. Unpatients-Why Patients Should Own Their Medical Data. Nature Biotechnology, 33(9):921–924, September 2015.

ownership of health data in the USA is actually playing a role in blocking the sharing of data and consequently locking up the value we can generate from our health data as a society. Merely framing the discussion in terms of access to data helps the companies that currently own your data and does little for the consumer. If we want to unlock the value of health data, we need platforms for consumers to store and control their data while also exercising some form of return to individuals and society. This is the raison d'être of healthbank.

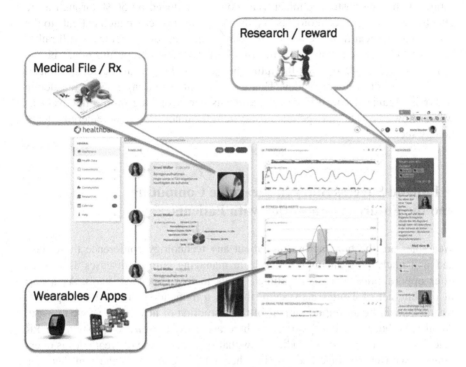

health bank Interface

The authors also discuss the potential revolutionary impact of bitcoin and blockchain on the current health data ownership models. Blockchain is a distributed cryptographic ledger platform that the cryptocurrency bitcoin is built upon. Blockchain enables greater security for data transactions and has potential applications for envisioning a new, more citizen-centric way of storing health, genomic, and financial data. One of the problems many health systems have, especially in the US context, is the lack of a unique identifier for every patient. Due to a Byzantine political process, this is currently a taboo subject in the US government. The lack of a unique identifier adds to the confusion in health informatics and possible safety issues and misidentification of patients. Blockchain could potentially provide a default solution to this problem while also maintaining high standards of privacy and security. At healthbank, we are actively involved in assembling some of the best minds on clinical research and Blockchain to position ourselves to play an important intermediary role in providing this type of service to citizens around the world and hopefully change the current ownership model of health data while incentivizing medical research and the pharmaceutical sector's transition to a "beyond the pill" paradigm.

Another component of the transition to a new "beyond the pill" business model for the pharmaceutical sector is the use of wearables and mobile applications that can be used in both clinical trials and disease management. There are some estimates that the costs of clinical trials could be reduced by 50 % through more effective use of these technologies and data analytics that can match patients to the appropriate clinical trials better. Yet the current market for wearables is still rather primitive. For insights into what the future of wearable computing might be we can see many signals of what the future holds by looking at the sector in Finland and move beyond Silicon Valley. This is a story of rethinking how the academic sector is organized and different departments can cooperate more effectively as well as how to create a cooperative ecosystem for innovation in an emerging technology sector.

A Finland Success Story in Wearable Computing and the Future of Innovation with Patients

Wearables are the buzz across just about any technology conference these days and will likely play an important role in managing chronic diseases as well as offer opportunities to conduct clinical trials in less expensive ways. As a part of the Internet of Things ecosystem, there is a tremendous amount of hope that wearables will be an important part of the disruption of healthcare as we know it. Amidst the buzz and hype, however, there are many reasons to question the PR machine behind the buzz as studies show that sustainable use of wearables is questionable with the average user tossing their latest wearable on the junk heap on their desks after 3–4 months. A lot of data is "dressed up with no place to go," that is, in apps or silos with few user-friendly tools to help users make sense of the data. This represents the old way of thinking about data capture which fails to leverage the value of data and engage patients in a more robust way. It is clear we are in the early days of wearable computing making inroads into improving health outcomes or quality of care. Yet, even skeptics admit that the future of healthcare is likely going to have wearables and data analytics as a central component of managing one's health and fitness. But what might that future look like?

If Malcolm Gladwell's observation that you need 10,000 h of practice to become an expert holds true, Finland undoubtedly has the highest number of wearable computing experts in the world, as Christian Lindholm of Koru Lab and HealthSpa, two Helsinki-based organizations focused on catalyzing innovation in the wearables arena, explains. Few observers of the emerging wearables market realize that Finnish entrepreneurs and technologists have been in this business for more than 30 years. That is just a year less than Apple. From heart rate monitor maker Polar Electro (http://www.polar.com/en), to the maker of one of the most important sources of innovation in battery design for wearables Suunto (https://en.wikipedia.org/wiki/Suunto), Finnish companies have been innovating in this space for well over a decade and also have a similar university–industry nexus similar to what we find in Silicon Valley. As the digital world fragments, the Finns unite and build bridges across the silos. Aalto University combined the premier design, engineering, and business schools to better support an innovative economy for Finland. Combine this with the University of Helsinki's reputation in public health and medicine and one finds a pretty robust academic test bed for innovation in digital health. Many will point to the demise of Nokia in recent years as perhaps indicating a weakness in the "culture of innovation" in Finland, but that fear may be misplaced. Many of the engineers from Nokia who lost jobs in recent years left with some intellectual property and a substantial severance package. Often this was just enough to launch a new start-up. Some of the older technology companies that are not focused on wearables have been around long enough to have alumni who have launched their own start-ups as well. What one encounters is an emerging innovation hub for one of the technologies that is predicted to become a $70 billion dollar market by 2024 by IDTechEx (http://www.idtechex.com/research/reports/wearable-technology-2015-2025-technologies-markets-forecasts-000427.asp).

HealthSpa: Launching the Next Generation of Wearables, and Globally

In 2012, Lindholm and partners launched HealthSpa (http://www.healthspa.fi), a health & happiness ecosystem to accelerate innovation in the health, wearables, and Internet of Everything computing domain where Finland has developed a comparative advantage in talent. Open innovation is the key word here. Early on they recognized that one of the problems in the digital health and wearables space is the silos within the ecosystem and that breaking down the silos between these companies and building opportunities for collaboration would help grow business opportunities for everyone. You can now find Beddit (http://www.beddit.com), the sleep sensor company working with Wellmo and PulseON (http://www.pulseon.fi), two data analytics companies, collaborating to offer feedback loops to users to improve sleep outcomes. These collaborations help the younger start-ups build up a customer base. This makes even more sense from the perspective of a small country that needs to build links to external markets to become financially sustainable.

HealthSpa includes both early stage start-ups and some of the more mature companies that have been designing wearables and related technologies for the past decade or more. Suunto has been developing dive computers, heart rate monitors, and other wearable technologies since 1997 with the Spyder watch diving computer. Their first GPS on the wrist the G9 was introduced in 2004 and they can claim ownership of the innovations that have extended the battery life of GPS devices from 8 h a decade ago to nearly 80 h in 2014. On the algorithm side, Firstbeat (http://www.firstbeat.com) develops heart rate variability algorithms that can be used to inform behaviors that mitigate stress or improve fitness. Formed in 2002 their products are now found in Garmin, Samsung, Suunto, and Bosch devices and have been used for professional athletes as well as occupational health applications for workplace wellness. Omegawave (http://www.omegawave.com), another company focusing on the algorithmic side of wearables, offers performance management software for athletes and teams to optimize performance based on the data gathered from ECGs, for example. UnderArmour (http://www.underarmour.com) recently conducted a competitive analysis of technologies in this space and Omegawave came out on top of the competition. Their technology was originally used in Russia and the USA bought back to Finland for consumerization and now includes clients such as the US Navy Seals, professional soccer teams, Olympians, and Seattle Seahawks. Heia Heia (http://www.heiaheia.com) also provides insights into the ways that data and design are likely going to work in the space in coming years. They have several years; worth of activity log data for everyday activities such as house cleaning and walking with the dog, which seems to be the 5th most done activity logged. One of the gaps in the current wearables space is insights on actual use of the devices that can lead to insights on why sustainability of use is so low. These activity logs may unearth a number of opportunity spaces for designers in the future. Heia Heia provides a service that is increasingly common-activity trackers linked to apps that can utilize various gamified or motivational modules to improve health outcomes in employee wellness programs. Already deployed in 140 countries, they may not be well known in the USA but include one of the largest fitness chains in Europe as a client. Heia Heia also demonstrates the power of collaboration within the local ecosystem. Hintsa Performance was developed by neurosurgeon Aki Hintsa, the senior physician for Finland's Olympic Committee, to aggregate data from neurological tests and through tracking sleep and other vital signs that can indicate general fitness and performance levels of athletes. Formula One racing team, McLaren, has been using the system to monitor Formula One drivers for years and finds it one of the most important forces behind selecting drivers who will compete in any given week. Heia Heia and Hintsa Performance are now collaborating to digitalize the service for a much wider customer base in the coming years.

One application that is currently focused on the fitness market and the posture of athletes may have many occupational health applications for those of us stooped over desks all day. MyonTec (http://www.myontec.com), listed by the New York Times (http://www.nytimes.com/interactive/2012/06/03/magazine/innovations-issue.html?_r=0) in 2012 as one of the innovators likely to change the future, utilizes a wide range of sensors found in many other fitness applications with the addition of sensors that monitor muscle load and posture. These sensors can do gait analysis, muscle training monitoring, analysis of movement disorders, and analysis of form in various activities. Users of the new Adidas wearables and smart watches might note that Metawatch and Elektrobit are two Finnish firms that are involved in a joint venture with Adidas wearables.

Koru Lab, Breaking the Mold for Interface Design and Wearables

Lindholm's own company, Koru Lab (koru means "jewelry in Finnish), and its trajectory over the two short years of its existence are an interesting case study in what may become of wearables in the next phase of innovation. Asked by a major technology platform to come up with the "killer app" for wearables, Lindholm spent a year working on an answer to this question and decided it was too early to frame the question in this manner. Instead, after thinking about the big challenge on the radar right now, curve fatigue or lack of sustainable engagement, a number of questions emerged from how to convey data collected via wearables and what new representational paradigms beyond the medical model could emerge to user-interface design for wearables. Also, how to move the price point down while maintaining a smooth iPhone-like experience on a microcontroller is a big technical issue. If devices have to be worn 24/7, they have to be beautiful, small, fast, and their battery cannot run out halfway through the second day. The current market for wearables is bifurcating with those devices that run on a microcontroller versus those that run on a CPU. This has profound implications for users and business models based on the traditional hardware and software paradigm where the manufacturer maintains control over the user interface. Just take a look at Apple and the degrees of freedom a user has in modifying the device, Zero. Koru has developed an incredibly small and flexible platform that runs on XML leveraging the SVG standard, not Java. This makes it easy to adopt by anyone familiar with HTML5. The most unique property is that any manufacturer can design their own experience from a set of more than 60 readymade components. This turns the traditional hardware and software model on its head by allowing manufacturers and even users to modify the device. Koru is the software platform that glues the technology and fashion industry together. Fashion meets technology, but with much more under the hood than meets the eye. Users will be able to modify the device to match outfits in the same manner you can change shoes based on the weather. Their devices can also run across Apple, Google, Samsung, and Microsoft's platforms. This is a big deal when you look at the global market and preferences across regional markets where some companies and consumers may not want to be tied to Google or Apple, for example.

Koru and HealthSpa have both attracted the attention of large Asian investors who sense the growing need for scalable digital health technologies over the next decade. China has over 10,000 villages that over the next decade will be virtually emptied of inhabitants under seventy. Telemedicine, sensors, and wearables are likely going to play a major role in providing remote healthcare opportunities for both the government and the consumers whose families are dispersed geographically. These large investors are taking note because this innovation cluster is likely going to have a major impact in how we think about wearables, health, and the business of hardware and software in the future. While we hear a lot these days about software eating the world, we may be on to something a bit different here.

Lindholm refers to "omni-platforms" that will emerge as the big players such as Google, Samsung, Apple, and Microsoft offering linked hardware and software services. Design and fashion loom large but need to be linked to a data service or as one Frog Design lead has commented, "design may include algorithms wrapped in nice shiny boxes in the future." Our current approach to serving up medical data in pretty graphs will need to migrate more into the realm of service design where products are merely avatars for an underlying data service. A glimpse of where this is going can already be detected in Suunto where the community and hobbyist have published 10,000 different apps, and another 5000 that are implemented for the individual. This is mass customization for the twenty-first century. These technological innovations when combined with the social technology of social supports, peer pressure, and behavioral economics-driven design and coaching engines are where we may see the wearables market going in the coming years. The Finns use of open innovation models to bridge the silos across an incredibly fragmented race to the market that we find in other parts of the globe, may make for a powerful test bed for wearables to actually live up to the hype.

Returning to Diabetes and the Concept of "People Powered Healthcare"

We began this chapter with a look at how patients have been self-organizing to create social supports and play a more active role in the research process through sharing data with clinical researchers. Our overview of healthbank demonstrates another aspect of platform creation that can support this overall move into incentivizing participation in research and rethinking ownership of health data away from the traditional model where hospitals and health IT companies own the patient's data. An important tool in this emerging network of people and things is the growing role of wearables and new zones of innovation and practices that may drive the next generation of wearable technology that can become more user friendly, provide better feedback to users in a way that can sustain engagement. There is another piece of this puzzle that could be brought into play with the components described above that addresses the social infrastructure of communities and innovation in healthcare delivery or just the production of good health, but outside of the traditional focus on medical care.

We now turn to the experience of the UK and an innovative approach to addressing chronic diseases and aging in place that the UK-based think tank NESTA developed from 2011–13. The People Powered Health program offers a valuable tool and way of thinking about design and co-creation in health that could be pulled together with the platforms and networks listed above to create innovative ecosystems of cooperation that are capable of generating new technologies, but most importantly, better health outcomes at lower price points.

The People Powered Health (PPH) program was launched in England in spring 2011 with a call for ideas. In total 106 teams applied and after a three-stage selection process, six teams from across England took part in the program. The local teams were each awarded a £100,000 grant and provided with a range of non-financial support to develop their capacity in fields such as co-production, service design, business case development and commissioning. We established a peer network between the teams to enable them to learn from one another as well as from external experts.

So what makes the People Powered Health approach?

The People Powered Health approach offers a vision for a health service in which:

- the health and social care system mobilises **people** and recognises their assets, strengths and abilities, not just their needs.
- the ability to live well with long-term conditions is **powered** by a redefined relationship, a partnership of equals between people and healthcare professionals
- the **health** and care system organises care around the patient in ways that blur the multiple boundaries between health, public health, social care and community and voluntary organisations

This vision is grounded in innovations that have emerged in health and social care over the last 20 years. It demands an urgent effort to make those innovations a normal part of our health and care systems. This will require a new balance between health provision for people, active health management by people, and mutual support with people.

The NHS in England could realise savings of at least £4.4bn a year if it adopted these People Powered Health innovations that involve patients, their families and communities more directly in the management of long term health conditions. These savings are based on the most reliable evidence and represent a 7 per cent reduction in terms of reduced A&E attendance, planned and unplanned admissions, and outpatient admissions.[2]

In a way, we can think about the NESTA approach as a "People as Infrastructure" approach to producing better health outcomes. Most of our digital health conversations focus purely on the technology components and data analytics that can drive change but neglect the so-called soft components. We talk a lot these days about patient engagement but in most cases this is lip service or a marketing slogan to go along with the latest trend in health IT. To add substance to the marketing slogans, we need to build more robust methodologies and take advantage of co-creation in the actual development of technology tools further upstream versus the traditional way of rolling out new technologies in the name of patient "empowerment" and "engagement" with a wish and a prayer assuming that the technology will play the magical role of making these things happen.

The PPH program is heavily focused on co-production of services and how peer-to-peer networks and co-design methodologies can be used in conjunction with rethinking of where and how care is delivered. Some of the examples used over the years included:

- A good case study of redesign is NeuroResponse (http://launchpad.youngfoundation.org/node/252); a social enterprise incubated by the Young Foundation's Launchpad (http://launchpad.youngfoundation.org/) that addresses the unmet

---

[2]http://www.nesta.org.uk/project/people-powered-health#sthash.rPqW223E.dpuf.

needs of patients with neurological disorders through the use of existing tele-communications infrastructures so that more patients can receive treatment at home, that is, moving from an acute care model to community care. The cost of a diagnosis of MS currently costs the system £17,000 per person or a total of £400 million of which the majority is for in-patient, hospital-based care. Telemedicine has the potential to save millions.

- The Expert Patient program (http://www.expertpatients.co.uk/) is another example of how self-care is being used to improve outcomes and patient satisfaction. Hospital admissions have been reduced by 50 % and visits to GPs reduced by between 40 and 69 %.
- Community-based initiatives tend to be better for behavioral change than top-down approaches. The Knowsley Primary Care Trust (http://www.invmeduk.com/nhs-health-checks/articles/nhs-health-checks---knowsley-health-and-well-being-partnership-71/) created a partnership for well-being that focuses on cardiovascular disease prevention at the community level and works through pubs, bingo halls, and shopping centers. The result has been a 28 % reduction in cancer morbidity rates and 32 % decrease in smoking.
- Well London (http://www.london.gov.uk/welllondon/) is a consortium of health, environmental, education, and arts organizations that invests in community projects for health behavioral change. This includes projects like Healthy Spaces that transforms open spaces into greener, more attractive places. Community mental health is one of the focus areas.
- Transforming Innovation: Perhaps the most difficult challenge is changing the way organizations think about innovation. The US public health sector is in dire need of this change in mindset. Getting funders AND organizations to take risks, experiment, move beyond dated ways of thinking about technologies and community is a challenge. One of the platforms they have used in the UK is Patient Opinion (http://www.patientopinion.org.uk/default.aspx), a platform that enables users of the NHS to provide feedback and develop networks of user citizens to provide the essential feedback that innovators within the system can use to improve services.
- Open Innovation for behavioral change: The Big Green Challenge (http://www.biggreenchallenge.org.uk/) is another initiative designed by NESTA focusing on climate change and how communities can reduce their carbon emissions. The program is essentially a platform that crowdsources ideas for innovative strategies and provides awards for the best proposals. The concept has been extended into the obesity/diabetes space through the Healthy Community Challenge Fund (http://www.dh.gov.uk/en/Publicationsandstatistics/Publications/DH_085328) to test and evaluate ideas that make activity and healthier food choices easier.

The underlying business case for the PPH approach was relatively inexpensive and ranged from approximately $150–700 per patient annually. NESTA has published a number of case studies and an overview of the overall business case for co-production of healthcare delivery.

From these components, we can also imagine how health data platforms, patient networks, and wearables (and/or sensors) may be assembled in the future to manage chronic conditions. Some of the scenarios envisioned by NESTA include the following:

- **Health Knowledge (Data) Commons**: With greater sharing of knowledge and improvements in biometric authentication and security, we may see greater transparency in how data are used and be able to more clearly see how it benefits others as well as receive feedback on how our own actions impact our health and the populations. If we drive our cars more, for example, we may worsen our own asthma as well as others. Wearables that can connect to platforms enable us to track data in more sensitive ways and encrypted but also see the data in aggregation or in analyzed form for our neighborhood, city, or region, for example.[3]
- **Health Data Markets**: Markets for personal health data emerge where the citizen maintains control and can bargain and barter for new products and services with their own data. Data for special conditions become more valuable and citizens can negotiate prices. Higher-quality wearables can authenticate and certify the reliability of your personal health data set.[4]
- **Health Data Provenance Systems**: Privacy breaches damage trust and citizens begin to set up their own provenance systems for health data that encourage sharing. This is where cooperative structures such as healthbank could also play a role as the Consumer Reports for health data provenance, accuracy, insurance, and financial transactions.[5]
- **Health Data Markets Explode**: When people realize the value of their health data, they find the means and devices to track and integrate many types of data and explore the meanings and analytics. Machine learning tools become more user friendly and enable both individual and collective analytics commons and cooperatives. Investment of your data in the market is automated.[6]
- **Surveillance Fears**: People are becoming distrustful of how data analytics can be used against them or without their consent, security breaches are increasing, and engagement with wearables is weak because users are not receiving useful feedback that can engage behavioral change. Devices such as Medi-Bloc have emerged to block tracking and collection of personal data due to the fears listed above. Devices such as Medi-Bloc emerge to block tracking and collection of personal data.[7]
- **Co-produced Service Society Emerges**: Networks of citizens–patients have digital infrastructures to enable co-created/produced services to proliferate and devices to support the underlying analytics and communications needed to

---

[3]http://www.nesta.org.uk/health-knowledge-commons-innersense.

[4]http://www.nesta.org.uk/personal-data-ecosystem-medihex.

[5]http://www.nesta.org.uk/health-system-shutdown-analogue.

[6]http://www.nesta.org.uk/data-makers-cumulus.

[7]http://www.nesta.org.uk/still-nation-medibloc.

coordinate care, provide transparency and incentivize data sharing. New wearables help people to engage in peer-to-peer support programs that have feedback
loops to technology companies and designers.[8]

- **Blockchain-enabled health records**: Blockchain (distributed, cryptographic,
  transaction ledger that bitcoin is built upon) matures and becomes the standard
  for storing encrypted health data and serves as the underlying infrastructure for
  distributed, peer-to-peer systems of support as well as the lynchpin of the health
  data economy that rewards sharing of data for the collective good. Healthcoins
  reward data sharing and peer-to-peer healthcare delivery programs and are used
  as payment for health services. A mature healthbank has become a platform in
  the true sense of the word that offers transparency in health data transactions
  and the foundations for robust data sharing while putting citizens in control and
  providing a socially responsible way to use data ethically but also drive innovation in wearables, sensors, and new health services.

I have taken the scenarios offered by NESTA and mashed them up with the ideals
behind our company healthbank, to show how we can envision a more innovative
economy based on data sharing with greater citizen control and through the use
of innovative wearables. We also see that no single technology or business model
alone can realize a better future but assemblages of different approaches, policies, and platforms when outfitted with the tools for cooperation may lead to more
effective uses of data in the future while still protecting privacy and security. A
lead role for patients as active participants in shaping these futures will be necessary and later in this book we discuss the potential for networks of patients and
their data to influence policy innovation as well as technology innovation. A key
piece in this future we have not discussed is the growing importance of algorithmic ethics. As more parts of the health system become automated and machine
learning tools proliferate off of our data sets, we will need to be vigilant in
addressing how new forms of discrimination and inequality may emerge from the
reliance on algorithms and develop policy tools and business practices to avoid
these cases.

---

[8]http://www.nesta.org.uk/health-and-care-system-alt.

Chapter 3
Rise of the e-Patient and Citizen-Centric Public Health

Jody Ranck

In the early 2000s as Google went from a Stanford graduate student project to becoming a verb we began to notice something interesting happening with search and health care. More and more people were using the Web to find information about health and how to manage their conditions. A mere six months after Google acquired YouTube in late 2006 we were discussing technology and health trends at the Institute for the Future and realized that we needed to do devote some major research time to understanding how consumers and patients were creating YouTube channels to share health information and knowledge. The new Web 2.0 platforms, search and YouTube, were beginning to change the way people managed health conditions and sought care. This was about the time that Matthew Holt coined the term "Health 2.0" on his healthcare blog, and the first conferences began popping up to tout these new media channels and their impact on health care.

At IFTF we had developed a framework to understand the new information ecology of resources that patients were mobilizing to manage their own health and their families. We called the framework the "Personal Health Ecology," and it included technologies, information sources, products, providers, activities, and even places—each of these categories had been exploding in recent years and we sought to use ethnographic data to understand how different demographic groups were cobbling together a loose patchwork of sources to improve their health and wellness (Fig. 3.1).

J. Ranck (✉)
Health Bank, Ranck Consulting, Ram Group, Washington D.C., USA
e-mail: jody@ranckconsulting.com

© Springer International Publishing Switzerland 2016   43
J. Ranck (ed.), *Disruptive Cooperation in Digital Health*,
DOI 10.1007/978-3-319-40980-1_3

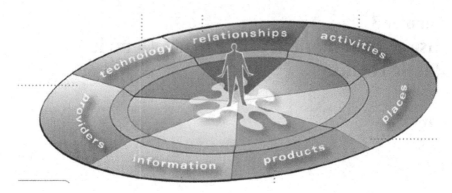

Fig. 3.1 Personal Health Ecologies. *Source* Institute for the Future (http://www.iftf.org/uploads/media/SR_876A_Personal_Health_Ecologies.pdf)

Since the 1960s the traditional biomedical model of health care had been shifting to a more diverse perspective that integrated a wider range of physicians and healers and had worked to diminish many of the traditional biomedical hierarchies, although they still exist. The established medical order had been changing as a generation caught up in the social movements of the 1960s had challenged established social orders on many fronts. The meaning of health had broadened to encompass things such as spirituality and wellness, for example. Yoga, massage, traditional Chinese medicine, and other therapeutic modalities were increasingly becoming mainstream, and health had steadily shifted to mean more than just the absence of disease. This was when broader perspectives on public health also took hold and we began looking at the built environment and the design of cities as factors in driving health outcomes.

Now with the rise of Web 2.0 tools and new media technologies the pluralization of medicine and health began to accelerate. These platforms do not automatically overturn or completely revolutionize health and medicine as some advocates suggest. We can find many of the same hierarchies and influences here. But one important shift has been the way that the internet and increasingly the mobile phone are democratizing health and medical information. You no longer need exclusive access to a major medical hospital or university library to access a great deal of health and medical information, although the current business model for academic journals still remains a major firewall for access to information outside of projects focusing on open access to health journals.

One of the challenges that the dramatic growth in health care spending and broadening definition of health created was an acceleration of the fragmentation of the overall health economy. More providers, more information, more products, more channels—this created a frightening situation for many healthcare providers and physicians. We began to hear more talk of patients showing up with reams of printouts from Google searches on people's conditions and demands for new therapies and drugs. This was the early days of a global shift in how patient groups were thinking about access as well. Act Up had catalyzed a great deal of activism in the 1980s–1990s around HIV and access to care, research dollars and the rights of those infected with HIV. The Genetic Alliance had formed numerous patient groups around genetic disorders and created lobbying groups and patient groups. In South Africa, the Treatment Action Campaign had taken on major pharmaceutical companies and the established intellectual property regime to fight for lower prices for life-saving HIV therapies in lower income countries. Anthropologists began talking of an emerging biological citizenship that captured how patient groups, on the basis of shared biological and biomedical experiences, could form and demand new rights within national and global contexts. The early days of these movements their technological arsenal typically included email and activist campaigns at major health conferences and national events. This was the pre-Facebook era.

Now, jump ahead a few years and the rise of many-to-many platforms such as Facebook, Twitter and patient-driven platforms such as PatientsLikeMe, TuDiabetes, MedHelp and the virtual explosion of Health 2.0 and the ability for patients to discover and connect to others sharing similar experiences has changed dramatically. We are now smack dab in the middle of the digital biocitizenship arena, and this is going to have a dramatic impact on health and medicine in the coming years. Patients now have an almost endless number of tools at their immediate disposal. If anything, the challenge is how to find the right ones for the right person and sort the snake oil salesmen from the information that is truly helpful.

The Emergence of the e-Patient: e-Patient Dave

Dave deBronkart, otherwise known as e-Patient Dave, is now a fixture in the connected health world due to his inspiring activism on behalf of patients struggling with the healthcare system, particularly those with life-threatening diseases. A former high-tech executive[1] has been a keen observer of technological changes and their impact on people's lives as they navigate the health system. For many years he had played an active role in online communities on Compuserv. In 2007, just as the Health 2.0 movement was getting started he was diagnosed with Stage IV kidney cancer which has a median survival rate of 24 weeks post-diagnosis. While receiving treatment at Boston's Beth Israel Deaconness Hospital he began utilizing the Web to optimize his treatment and mobilize his social network to assist in his care. One of the early health bloggers, he became quite adept at exploiting the utility of online patient forums such as the Association of Cancer Online Resources and other cancer-related Web sites, even writing on the hospital blog as "Patient Dave." Eventually he recovered from the kidney cancer and re-named himself as

---

[1]His personal story is captured on his blog: http://epatientdave.com/about-dave/#.ULZsgzn6bDo.

"e-Patient Dave" and launched a post-recovery blog that could serve as a resource for others in a similar health predicament.[2]

One particular event gave deBronkart pause and insights into the current state of dysfunction of health technology and some insights on what needed to be done to improve patient care. In 2009 he decided to download his medical record data from the hospital into Google Health, a personal health record that Google closed down in 2011. Much to his surprise the data from his health record were full of errors: exaggerated diagnoses, false medication warnings, erroneous laboratory and radiology results, and so on. Many of the errors were due to the use of billing data, and the news of deBronkart's experience soon ended up as front-page news in the Boston Globe because EMRs were a hot button topic in 2009 as the stimulus package was being crafted and had an economic incentive to promote the use of electronic records.

By 2009 the term "e-Patients" had become more widespread in health technology circles and we had seen some very interesting examples of other patients using blogs and online tools for important advocacy issues. Prominent diabetes blogger, Amy Tenderich, author of Diabetes Mine, had notoriously spoken out about the poor design of insulin pumps and wondered out loud on her blog why diabetics do not have their own Steve Jobs who could create a more user-centric design for the pumps. The result was a major San Francisco-based design firm picked up on the challenge and soon created a more innovative pump. This further demonstrated the power of online communities for mobilizing and advocating for solutions to their unmet needs.

e-Patient Dave has continued his efforts and speaks widely to this day about a whole host of e-health issues that includes the need for better interoperability and design of digital health tools that could enhance the patient experience. The activist voice has been quite central in the policy debates over the creation of "Meaningful Use" criteria that are an important part of the health IT regulatory environment in the coming years, namely around the aspects that have to do with patient engagement with health IT and the design of technologies that are more patient-centric. When some quarters of the technology sector have resisted these efforts, deBronkart is a prominent spokesperson on patients' behalf.

Moving Beyond the Spokesperson to the Mainstream e-Patient

The notion of the e-Patient took hold in an era of e-governance, e-health and expanding use of electronic and information technologies across the economy. However, the interesting thing about the patients using Web 2.0 platforms for health care is that the "e" evolved to take on a rather different meaning. These

---

[2]http://en.wikipedia.org/wiki/Dave_deBronk.

were patients demanding greater voice in the healthcare system and in determining how health technologies evolved. This was not about a passive audience awaiting health technology innovation from above, much the way "innovation" in health care had happened in the past. After all, it is no easy feat to become a biotechnologist or physical chemist developing the next-generation drug. The algorithmic revolution and how it played out in the Web 2.0 world was one where the revolution was more about ease of use and empowering a do-it-yourself ethos. We are all familiar now with teenagers developing new software capable of doing things that previously took a PhD computer scientist to pull off in the 1990s. The ethos of Web 2.0 came together with some long-standing trends in the evolution of health and health care to shape the way health 2.0 was going to unfold. Notice the language here—Health 2.0 is most often spoken about as a "movement" not just a technological trend. Patients and what anthropologists would term "biocitizens" began using the "e" to mean "empowered" or "engaged" and making calls for participatory medicine.

This marks a shift from a very traditional physician–patient as well as public health–public relationship that, in the most stereotyped form, had those with the expertise working from a position of superiority in relationship to the patient/public. e-Patients and the participatory medicine community are calling for the health and medical professions to be in a different type of relationship or as a partnership in care. This is recognition that the devolution of health knowledge that information technologies are bringing about a transformation that is much deeper than what the notion of "disruptive technology" implies.

Italian philosopher of information, Luciano Floridi, has captured this fundamental shift in the information ecology quite well.[3] The current era is the era of the "Fourth Technological Revolution." The first revolution was the era of Copernicus and astronomy where how we came to think about the place of the Earth in the universe was overturned. Copernicus overthrew the Ptolemaic model that postulated the earth at the center of the universe. The second revolution was the result of Darwin's theory of evolution. Freud's insights into the nature of the unconscious launched the third scientific revolution. We are now in the fourth scientific revolution that was inspired by Alan Turing, the mathematician who helped develop the first computers. But this is more than just another disruptive technology like the iPhone, Floridi cautions. Information is becoming part of the environment. We see this in the internet of things and the way that mobiles can give us information in situ about the locations we inhabit. The embeddedness of information has created "infosphere" and rather than becoming the cyborgs from the Terminator, we are increasingly "inforgs." Beyond the terminology, this has implications for health, the body and can help explain the shift to engaged, participatory e-Patients as well.

For Floridi the information revolution has three primary effects—the creation of the transparent body, the shared body, and the socialized body. Digitalization

---

[3]http://www.youtube.com/watch?v=yJJzDPqy9-E.

of life has created each of these possibilities. If you have been paying attention to science and popular culture at all of late you will have noticed the proliferation of popular articles on the neurosciences that attempt to explain, well just about all human behavior, whether rightly or wrongly. What has fueled much of the growth in the neurosciences is the use of MRI scans and CT scans, especially fMRI. Increasingly all dimensions of the body can be rendered in digital images, hence the transparent body. These images and data can be shared as we have seen throughout this book, on platforms that enable the display of visual information. Now, once you can "see" the body, share the data about one's body, this opens up the opportunity to "socialize" the body in new ways. This gets back to the notion of biocitizenship and much of the activity we see where patients can now reach out and find others with similar experiences. Connected health also connects people. Connected health actually has a very profound meaning beyond just implying digital connectivity. We may not quite yet have the language for understanding all that is going on here, but we can see through the voices of those involved with the participatory medicine movement that the injection of patient voices is going to change how we think about health, the body, and medicine in the coming years.

Some social scientists have been wary of the rhetoric of the Quantified Self movement, and some of the discourse in the Health 2.0 world for basically extending the reach of biomedicine and "colonizing" people's lifeworlds with a language that may not be their own. Using sophisticated social theory that has been used to critique biomedicine and the biomedicalization of social problems in the past may have a place, but we are not convinced that this captures everything that is happening. Of course, these are still ongoing issues but it strikes us as too rote. While any emerging technology, especially when it comes to Silicon Valley and other major technopoles, can have a great deal of what they call the "political economy of hype and hope" behind it, we think there is something novel and important that bodes well for patients here. It is striking how patients and activists concerned with the shape of digital health are actively involved in the crafting of policy, injecting their voices into the design of technologies, and pushing health care in new directions.

Who Owns the Data? e-Patients and the Debates Over Privacy and Ownership

An interesting window into the future of policy and patient activism is through the issue of who controls the data collected on one's device. A front-page story in the *Wall Street Journal* on November 29, 2012, brought this message home. Innocuously entitled, "Heart Gadgets Test Limits of Privacy Laws on Health"[4] discusses the controversy that has arisen out of the realization that personal health

---

[4]http://online.wsj.com/article/SB10001424052970203937004578078820874744076.html.

data are becoming an asset for device makers, but patients often want to control how their health data are used. The article specifically focuses on the medical device manufacturer Medtronic, maker of pacemakers or defibrillator implants that collect data on one's heart. The way these implants work is to transmit data from the patient's body to a home monitor that can then transmit these data to a server housed by Medtronic. The data include information on heart rhythms and rates as well as information on the device performance. The patient's doctor can then log on to a Medtronic Web site to get a report on the data that have been collected. So far this is not that complicated.

Where we begin to see some possible friction points is in the following area. The article quotes a senior executive at Medtronic who publicly acknowledged that "data are the currency of the future." Across the digital health landscape, there is a race to collect data and develop new data analytics services that can help both patients and providers with care. This is a good thing and obviously holds the promise of bringing major improvements in the quality of care through personalization in the coming years. The challenge is that our policy frameworks have not kept apace of the technology developments and changes in the marketplace for data that these new technologies are creating. The bottleneck is that patients often do not have access to the data collected on their own bodies.

A device that just collects data and does not provide a therapy has different regulatory frameworks around it. Now we have the e-Patient phenomenon and patients demanding greater engagement and more participatory medical encounters wanting access to the data; we are rapidly approaching a policy bottleneck. The problem is that to make this happen from a device manufacturer perspective means designing a new platform that can handle streaming data in a format that patients can make sense of as well as Food and Drug Administration approval—a process that can take years. Doctors are in a quandary over whether patients could make adequate use of the raw data. In their support, we know that typical laboratory results are in a format that is challenging to interpret and this has become an area of a certain amount of entrepreneurial focus that would make the data more usable by patients. Other physicians feel that if it is patient data the patients should have access. Talk to folks in the e-Patient communities and the issue will be straightforward—patient data are the patient's data and they should have control over it. But in the case of medical devices, the data go to the medical device manufacturer that puts it beyond the scope of HIPAA's patient access requirements, as the WSJ article states.

One of the e-Patients, or what we might more accurately term, biocitizens, because he is exercising a right or claim within the healthcare system, to control his own data is Hugo Campo. The WSJ piece highlights his campaign to exert greater control and ownership over health data. Also the recipient of a Medtronic defibrillator, he prefers to frame this device just as one would any other tracking device on the market these days such as a Fitbit or Nike Fuel band. He has taken on Medtronic for access to his data and made some headway but not total access as he would prefer. As a self-proclaimed member of the Quantified Self movement, he also used a Zeo (a sleep tracking device manufacturer that was an early pioneer that also went out of business) and tracks his sleep, diet, and exercise. He has even taken his campaign to TED (http://www.youtube.com/watch?v=oro19-15M8k), the well-known forum for thought-provoking ideas and presentation, and pressed his case for his right to data. The "e" here in Campos's case could also mean "equipped" with devices and platforms for amplifying his message.

Control over one's data is becoming a major hot button issue. There is a serious trust issue in the civic sphere at large and the way that personal data are becoming monetized, or becoming a new economic asset as the World Economic Forum would have it. In early 2015, the issue of access to health data suddenly became a bigger political issue as the lack of interoperability and "data blocking" by EHR providers became a political issue in the halls of Congress while a nascent movement to catalyze e-Patients to demand their data from EMRs was launched under the "Get My Data" rubric. In the 1990s the hot button issue was genetic privacy and concerns that employers and health plans could use your genetic data against you. Today the types of data collected and the ease of collection as well as the overall market for data have all exploded at a rather dizzying pace and the hot button issues run the gamut of control and ownership to access and privacy. It is no wonder that policymakers are challenged to keep pace with the changes but now more than ever we need to wrap our heads around this and come up with some proactive responses to data politics. Privacy legislation such as HIPAA is reasonably good at preventing third parties from using health data in the ways that people imagine. But with sensors, mobile phones, apps, and medical devices that can come under different legal regimens there is plenty of room for maneuver in the overall digital health space. The WSJ article makes the valid point that if a patient downloads an iPhone app that is not a prescribed device or application there is no legislation to protect the patient's rights. Data in electronic medical records are protected by HIPAA and through enforcement activities of the Office of Civil Rights in the USA. Data breaches, under the new Health Information Technology for Economic and Clinical Health Act (HITECH), that affect more than 500 people must be reported to the Office for Civil Rights under the US Department of Health and Human Services. The OCR has created a "Wall of Shame" that lists healthcare companies that have had security and privacy breaches. In 2012 alone at least six organizations experienced breaches of records that involved one million or more records.[5] 2015 marked an even greater moment in the annals of hacking as several of the largest insurers in the country experienced hacking attacks that exposed the records of millions of patients.

A recent report authored by Jane Sarasohn-Kahn and published by the California Healthcare Foundation notes the growing economy of data in health care that goes well beyond the data in our health records.[6] The data exhaust from our retail purchases and everyday lives are being combined with our health data to create risk profiles. Risk has always been a central dimension of how insurance

---

[5]http://www.computerworld.com/s/article/9230028/_Wall_of_Shame_exposes_21M_medical_record_breaches.

[6]http://www.chcf.org/publications/2014/07/heres-looking-personal-health-info/.

companies operate, but the dramatic growth of data and the new rules of the road in post-Accountable Care Act or value-based systems means the risk burdens are shifting. The credit score used in finance is entering into the healthcare discourse where it also includes your financial situation as a proxy for your health status or health risk profile. In her study of health data, Sarasohn-Kahn points to the lack of transparency in how these data are being handled and we will increasingly need privacy laws that can keep up with the technology and business changes.

Now think about some of the innovations we discuss in this book such as passive monitoring through cell phone use. Passive monitoring allows researchers to obtain a window into one's social interactions and moods for example. These data can be extremely valuable in developing the next generation of prevention and behavioral change methodologies for everything from chronic diseases to medication adherence regimens. Employers are increasingly interested in a range of mobile wellness programs that can help them prevent illnesses in the workforce and save healthcare dollars. But these also raise the specter of "Big Brother" and an encroaching surveillance society. We can offer incentives such as lower health insurance premiums if people participate but for many individuals this is going to feel like Bentham's panopticon, but only exerting even more control as we enter into the world of nano-sensors and electronic tattoos that are in or on the body. This is why taking note of the changing idea of patients and biocitizens and how they can use modern communications tools to clear space within the system for their voices to be heard. New policy frameworks and technology tools that have privacy controls designed into the application in a user-centric fashion can help address the fears that some of these innovations may provoke.

e-Patient Networks

Some major funders in the healthcare arena have picked up on these trends and are actively funding ways to support networks of engaged patients who can collaborate with technology designers and healthcare providers to innovate in healthcare delivery. Perhaps the most influential foundation in this regard is the Robert Wood Johnson Foundation that developed an explicit approach for working with patients and laypersons to redesign some elementary aspects of health care. Think about it, what other field would tolerate customers sitting in an office for an hour to wait for an appointment like we do in health care. What other hyper-modern sector of the economy still relies on faxes and manual delivery of data from one vendor to another? Why do not we know the cost of services when we need to use the service or provider? In 2006 the RWJF launched Project Health Design to try out some experiments that could have the potential to change health care as we know it. Interdisciplinary teams of researchers, technologists, clinicians, and patients have been developing new tools to engage in better care and communicate with providers and caregivers.

One of the early experiments has been to address the issue of what kind of data belongs in a health record and not only has meaning for a physician but for the patient as well. Given the types of data we can collect on the cell phone, we can obtain a greater understanding of the everyday patterns of life and hopefully uncover beneficial insights that can improve care and outcomes, beyond just feeding fears of the surveillance society. The Project Health Design approach has been to find a way to record "observations of daily living" (ODLs) that include feelings, thoughts, behaviors, and environmental factors.[7] In effect what they are trying to do is create a more participatory personal health record that can improve both the science and art of the clinical encounter and build bridges between the patient and provider. This often gets lost in all of the discussion about electronic health records and digital health. We can see in efforts like this how the human dimension does not get lost in really innovative design processes and technology, design and human-centeredness can all come together in important ways.

Project Health Design also shows how data are not just raw facts but have a living breathing dimension around the meanings that people attach to experiences and how health care is produced. These are the things that will matter if we want to truly engage people in the health technologies of tomorrow. Health is increasingly produced—let us take that back—always has been produced primarily away from the clinic. What the doctor does in the doctor's office is a single data point, an episodic encounter. It is an essential and extremely important data point, but not the only data point that matters in what economists like to call the health production function. People's social worlds matter a lot, most physicians get this too. So the ODL approach can help inform new types of conversations and make it easier for all parties involved to obtain a better understanding of things like the social determinants of health—we know these are extremely important but the biomedical model and the nature of the clinical encounter often get in the way of physicians actually having the ability to include this in the practice of medicine.

A participatory process around the design of the next generation of personal health records is targeted to developing the features that have meaning for patients outside of the clinical setting but of relevance to both the clinician and patient. One of the expert patients that has played a major part of the RWJF efforts is a student at the University of California, Berkeley, who has spent over 10,000 h in hospitals as a patient with Crohn's disease, a disorder that affects 600,000 Americans.[8] Crohn's disease is an extremely painful inflammatory disease that affects the intestinal tract and can be life threatening. As a teenager Nikolai spent a great deal of time as a patient repeating the same information over and over to a number of different specialists throughout his hospital stays. The limitations of current EHR/PHRs were brought home when he participated in an experimental therapy that used hookworms to suppress the immune response and inflammation in his gut. His daily regimen got in the way as a student studying for final exams,

---

[7]healthit.hhs.gov/.../Brennan_Health_in_Everyday_Living.pdf.

[8]http://online.wsj.com/article/SB10001424052748703960004575427531544486778.html.

and he forgot to track his weight and energy levels. In the course of studying he had unknowingly become anemic and lost weight because the hookworms were drawing too much blood and the experimental therapy did not have the desired effect. A record that would have enabled him to track more of his daily regimen might have set off alarms earlier before the therapy had gone awry. It is insights such as these from engaged and wired patients that are feeding into the design process that will create a PHR that is more in tune with patients as well as providers. One of the most important outcomes of endeavors like this will be improvements in the quality of care when patient and provider can have more informed discussions based on the data collected.

The PHR can also be integrated with patient platforms where collectivities of like-minded patients can aggregate data or provide coaching to one another, advocacy, and a sense of community. While PHRs remain a rather obscure technology at the moment, they do hold potential if they can be designed from patient needs and connected to a wider ecosystem of tools and communities in a secure manner. Below is an illustration from the Aligning Forces for Quality program developed by RWJF with the explicit focus of harnessing the power of PHRs for patient empowerment (Fig. 3.2).

Aggregated records can also be anonymized and then mined for insights about the nature of disease and for finding cures as we will see in our case study of CureTogether. Increasingly patients can connect their tracking devices to their PHRs so weight, blood pressure, prescriptions, sleep, fitness, and nutritional data

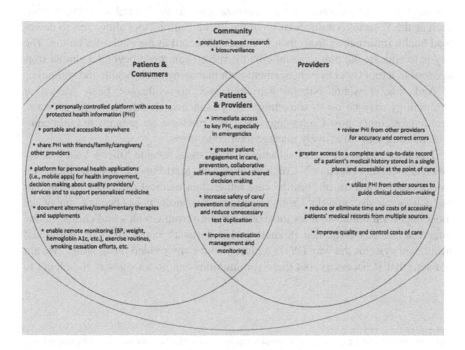

Fig. 3.2 Value of personal health records (*Source* AFQ Program)

What if we could learn from the collective experience of patients everywhere?

Top Medications			Top Diets			Top Supplements		
Remicade	★★★★	2180 people	No Beer	★★★★	1820 people	Vitamin B12	★★★★	1968 people
Prednisone	★★★★	3894 people	No Spicy Food	★★★★	1512 people	Vitamin D	★★★★	2446 people
Imuran	★★★	1948 people	No Dairy	★★★★	1547 people	Probiotics	★★★★	2381 people

Michael Weiss
West Orange, NJ
Multivitamin ★

Source Crohnology.com

can be stored and analyzed in data visualizations. At the federal level innovations such as the Veterans Affairs creation of the "Blue Button" tool allow vets to download health information from their VA medical record at the click of a button. The key is to educate the public about how the record can move beyond a simple storage tool to a tool for active engagement with managing one's health and wellness.

And this is where Nikolai Kurienko and his colleague Sean Ahrens at Crohnology may be on to something. They launched Healthy Labs (http://www.healthylabs.com/) (now Crohnology.com) as a platform for patients to build communities and tools to actively manage their conditions.

The start-up has also received interest from some notable Silicon Valley investors and incubators such as Y Combinator and the Start Fund. In a sense, these networks provide a form of "health" care rather than medical care. The two are not mutually exclusive, and the Crohn's platform, Crohnology, has become one of the most important online sources for those suffering from Crohn's and colitis. In one interview Ahrens is quoted predicting that software could supplant traditional healthcare systems the way DVDs replaced your corner video rental store.[9] We are not sure that is necessary, but these communities can go a long way in helping to

---

[9]http://www.fastcoexist.com/1680617/could-epatient-networks-become-the-superdoctors-of-the-future.

create a more distributed healthcare system that can improve the quality of care while not draining the nation's and households' bank accounts.

These are good examples of Luciano Floridi's socialized body or what we might want to call Open Health. This was another subject of a conference we sponsored at the Institute for the Future in 2007. We wanted to capture the potential for bringing into alignment the emerging trends around peer-to-peer health, open innovation, Web 2.0, the commons and cooperative business models. We will explore the intersections of some of these themes throughout the book, but we think what Floridi alludes to if we move from his emphasis on the body to health and wireless technologies as well as some of the health data practices we are beginning to see with greater frequency is a more open health system. Transparency is growing in importance and beginning to have an impact on more and more of the healthcare system. The e-Patients we talk about here are demanding more of it. Traditional notions of intellectual property are beginning to shift so that we can learn from open source software and open innovation platforms such as InnoCentive and cultures of sharing (data) to see new ways of doing things in health care.

e-Patients and Public Health

Many professions have their internal tribes and divisions, and medicine and health care are obviously not immune to the idea of different professional and ideological camps. One of the authors here is a physician with some public health training, the other a public health expert. We have both seen this play out in practice where public health views itself as the less hierarchical, more democratic, and populist profession. But we need to occasionally interrogate the assumptions supporting this. Public health has its own internal divisions between epidemiologists and community health activists, to name one example. But if we look at the public and the way they view public health, our profession often appears less hierarchical and democratic than we think When you think about the manner in which public health often appears in the news it should come as no surprise that mistrust of the profession is somewhat warranted. One week we hear that consuming more Vitamin D is going to protect you against cancer, next month it will increase your risk of cancer. Lifelong user of sunscreen, you got it, a study shows that it will not help you. You belong to a patient group and have been collecting and aggregating data from your tracking device and you want to present at a conference. Good luck, you do not have MPH or PhD after your name so the options have been limited for you to do a study and write it up for a peer-reviewed journal. But things are changing. For years one of us has been talking about health 2.0 and public health 2.0 at major health conferences and it is pretty much guaranteed that the first question from the audience of public health professionals is going to be focused on the corrupting influence of having non-professionals collect data and do research. However, the rise of citizen science initiatives that utilize mobile technologies, crowdsourcing platforms, gamification and other tools to harvest knowledge from non-professionals is beginning to change the traditional views of expertise. Public health has a tradition of popular epidemiology and community-based practice that can now be enhanced through engagement with open data platforms and these technologies to scale these initiatives in new ways.

If public health had been paying attention to the broader social and technology trends of the past 20 years or so they would have seen long ago that companies had begun opening up to ideas beyond their own walls. Open innovation and using ideas from lead users of their products is not as new as people think. This is a new way of thinking about design, and it needs to become part of the mainstream practice of public health. *More than participatory medicine, we need participatory health that can engage with the digital health ecosystem*. Rather than fearing the outside we need to embrace it. When I taught human rights and health at the University of California at Berkeley in the 1990s, I often used the work of Paul Farmer, the physician-anthropologist who has worked for decades in Haiti (and now Rwanda) to improve access to health care and life-saving medications. He also helped catalyze interest in teaching social medicine at Harvard Medical School. Social medicine brings public health insights on the social determinants into medical care. We have a tremendous opportunity to re-invigorate public health and social medicine with digital tools or what we would call digital social medicine.

The democratization of health knowledge, while not complete, is opening up opportunities to engage with communities and build civic apps that can make collective action around community health problems more effective. In the same manner that e-Patients are starting to take control of their own data and health records to improve the quality of care, citizens can use their own data plus public records and data collected by the government and create apps for mobiles and other devices to improve the health of their neighborhoods. Many will be doing this without public health expertise too.

One good example from urban planning is illustrative. As part of a 2012 Code for America fellowship, Matt Hampel and Prashant Singh developed a digital toolkit called LocalData (http://www.golocaldata.com) for community activists that helps people collect and manage place-based data. The kit helps people build surveys, collect data on mobiles or on paper and then export the data into a number of different formats that can be used to create visualizations. Users of the toolkit will be less dependent upon city planners to make sense of the data. People who know the most about the neighborhood and the data actually get to crunch the data.[10] The toolkit is already being used in Detroit to track urban blight. The founders have also created a new "civic start-up" called Amplify Labs that focuses on technology development for use at the local level.

---

[10]http://www.fastcodesign.com/1670954/localdata-an-app-that-helps-communities-do-their-own-urban-planning#1.

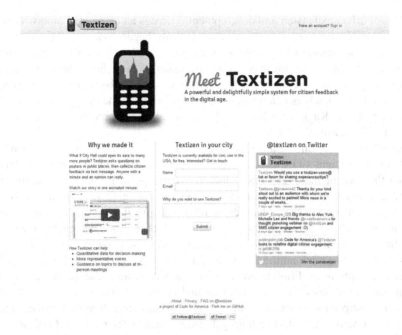

If you need funding for that civic tech project you can even crowdsource funding for your effort on Citizinvestor. Citizinvestor helps you find interesting public works projects that lack sufficient funding and one can donate small amounts of funding to support the cause. It is an interesting platform where we might be able to find ways to enhance engagement and ownership of local community health efforts, particularly in an era when funding is often being cut. The danger is that these types of platforms could be too heavily relied upon and this allows elected officials to let public health fall between the cracks. Code For America produced another interesting civic app called Textizen (http://www.textizen.com) that is a mobile app to "open the ears of City Hall" by asking questions on posters put up around the city that are essentially survey instruments about urban planning related questions.[11] These are generally simple yes or no question about things like transportation and other urban amenities. Neighborland (http://neighborland. com) is a similar mobile app developed by Tulane University, Rockefeller Foundation and Candy Chang, an urban designer, lets residents express what types of amenities they would like in their neighborhood but also has suggestions for how to actually implement the suggested projects.

Apps and data visualizations can sometimes go astray and be on the receiving end of engaged citizens and patients anger. A good example of this is when Stamen Design, an organization with a very good track record of developing powerful data visualizations worked with Trulia, the real estate search and information platform to build Trulia Hindsight (http://hindsight.trulia.com), that helps users see

---

[11]http://engagingcities.com/article/new-mobile-technology-solutions-offer-expanded-options-citizen-involvement.

patterns of urban expansion and development. There is an associated blog with the initiative and in one case residents of a community began attacking the visualization because it appeared as though their neighborhood was a missile target in a video game.[12] But there are many other examples of civic hackathons that have been bringing together communities, city officials, and programmers to identify unmet needs that hackers can develop new tools around. The data science crowdsourcing platform Kaggle has been used to create air quality prediction tools based on open EPA datasets for Chicago.[13]

OpenPlans.org is an organization that builds open source tools that can help create more efficient and inclusive local government. The whole concept is built around the idea of making it easier to take advantage of the information that is available and get the public more involved in city planning which tends to be a very top-down process. They have been involved with the creation of bike share apps in cities like Portland that have been innovators in urban design and creating a cycling culture that is both good for exercise and making the city greener. Place Pulse (http://pulse.media.mit.edu/) is a platform developed at MIT that crowd-sources perceptions of different urban areas as a way to study the manner in which urban perception has an impact on social and economic outcomes. The data can be used to help understand the connections between perception and crime, creativity or economic growth. Dr. Jeffrey Brenner formed the Camden Coalition of Healthcare Providers to collaborate around identifying the drivers of "super-utilizers" in the health system who account for most hospital emergency room admissions. The statistical methodology of cluster analysis was used from integrating billing data with community data to identify where the highest utilizers came from. Once the hot spots were identified, the causes of the trend could be identified and community-based approaches were used to bring the hospitals and medical care providers together with community organizations to address the problem. This is a good example of how medical systems can build effective collaborations beyond the clinic walls without boiling the ocean and losing sight of their mission.

Big data, urban planning, and health are likely to come together in interesting ways in the coming years. At the University of California, Berkeley, the Urban Systems Collaborative (http://urbansystemscollaborative.org/) unites different disciplinary perspectives such as urban planning, architecture, geography, environmental sciences, and health to study how cities actually work, develop metrics for data collection, and use design challenges and competitions for innovations that address citizen concerns about everything from the decline in privacy to the development of new services. While the collaborative does not engage directly in open data programs, their work intersects with the evolving landscape of open data as data can become an important connection between citizens and government. Open data can act as a catalyst for the public health version of the e-Patient as it pertains to engaged citizens getting more involved with urban planning and design issues

---

[12]http://www.greenplum.com/blog/topics/data-for-good/how-can-data-science-serve-the-public-good.
[13]http://www.kaggle.com/c/dsg-hackathon.

that are often carried out in top-down fashion. Andrew Barry refers to the increasing use of technology in society and the new roles of citizens in this environment as a new form of technological citizenship. What he means by this is that increasingly we will find it necessary to have a fairly sophisticated knowledge of technology to exercise one's rights and responsibilities as a citizen. This offers both an opportunity and a challenge. The sophistication of tools we have at our disposal offers greater insights into how cities actually work, where resources are allocated versus where they are needed most. We can obtain more nuanced understandings of the environmental drivers of health outcomes and so on. But on the other hand, even when technologies are made to be relatively user-friendly there will be communications and usability gaps that we will need to address. Data literacies are one area but gaps in access to mobile phones, for example, can have a major impact on equity.

There have been some interesting success stories at the city level over the past decade that are now in the process of becoming digitalized and hopefully even more participatory. One interesting international example is the use of participatory budgeting that took off in the Brazilian city of Porto Alegre in the late 1980s. In the years after the demise of the military dictatorship several community-based organizations (CBOs) began lobbying for more transparency at the municipal level, particularly in how local government funds were spent. The City of Porto Alegre has spent an average of $200 million per year on construction and city services. The participatory budgeting process divided the city into distinct neighborhoods where local assemblies were created where citizens could identify local priorities. The 16 districts of the city typically meet in January to begin the process of identifying sanitation, health, transportation, education, sports, and economic development priorities for their district. A series of meetings and an election for district representatives takes place and over a period of about 2–3 months the assemblies discuss the technical issues for the local priorities that have been identified by the assembly. In an average year about 50,000 residents out of the total population of 1.5 million participate directly in the process. A plenary group works on finalizing the city budget which can receive suggestions from the city council but not be changed by the council. The Mayor has the power to veto the budget but to date this has yet to occur.[14] The process has actually proven to be quite effective at improving sewer and water connections, improving educational outcomes as well as making an important contribution to public health outcomes. Since the program's launch in 1989 Porto Alegre has even become a major magnet for large corporate investments despite the history of very active trade unions that actually helped launch the process. One of our authors (Jody) attended a major conference on participatory budgeting that took place at the University of California, Berkeley, in the late 1990s, and it was reported that companies found that absenteeism rates and general satisfaction with life in the city had improved dramatically making it an attractive location for business. In fact, several major business newspapers had named Porto Alegre as one of the top cities to do

---

[14]http://en.wikipedia.org/wiki/Participatory_budgeting.

business in. In spite of this, one of the shortcomings of the participatory budgeting process was that in times of high unemployment the process had little impact on reducing unemployment for low-income residents. Nevertheless, the success of the Porto Alegre experiment has resulted in the adoption of similar efforts worldwide and a global network that develops tools to help other communities adopt the process.[15]

What all of these examples have in common is that they are creating conditions for more participatory design and co-production of the city. This is an important trend that will ultimately play a growing role in public health and could be an opportunity for more medical and mainstream public health programs to extend their reach through place-based applications and data science to both enhance our understanding of the role of place in health outcomes and to engage in this type of design process to build social innovations that can influence the design of local communities.

e-Patients and the Future of Health and Policy

We provide this example as a reminder that there is more work to do beyond the technology and that institutional and policy innovations need to complement the technology innovation. A great deal of the activism by e-Patients and citizens engaged in open data or participatory budgeting processes is about inserting patient and citizen voices into the technology and policy contexts so that they can play an active role in determining technology and policy trajectories of the future. The era of top-down, technologist, or policy wonk knows best is coming to a close. In Europe the gap between health technology and e-Patients was explicitly acknowledged in a recent European Commission eHealth policy action plan. The European Commission is the executive body for the European Union and recommends legislation, upholds treaties (when the European Union goes after Microsoft or Google for anti-trust issues it is through the European Commission), but have recently issued an eHealth Action Plan[16] that, even in the title, puts patients front and center for their overall digital health strategy. The approach is to provide legal support for start-ups while also engaging with the citizenry and healthcare workers to find ways to enhance the adoption of digital health tools for fear that the field is moving too slowly given the health challenges Europe faces in the current economic crisis.

As the digital health field matures there are likely going to be many friction points as patients, citizens and caregivers increasingly insert their views into policy and technology development debates. Many previously unheard of tensions points will arise as the technologies are adopted and used in new ways, often in

---

[15]http://www.participatorybudgeting.org.

[16]http://europa.eu/rapid/press-release_IP-12-1333_en.htm.

unforeseen ways. Caregiving roles that we are currently unaware of may come to the forefront, particularly as the medical home grows in popularity. Being sick or trying to avoid becoming sick takes a lot of work, particularly if you are taking care of a sick relative or family member. As we mentioned earlier, this is also costly. There are also new roles emerging in the digital health space: Telehealth requires tele-nurses, tele-doctors, and so on to support more distributed care. Software for workforce management commonly used in the telecommunications arena is ideal for filling in these gaps. In this soup of technologies and people things such as privacy, participation, and responsibility will take on many meanings; many meanings beyond what policy requirements and technology developers currently use. When does distributed care and "consumer-driven" health care become too burdensome? Who is paying for what and how does the drive toward greater transparency in quality of care enter into patients' and citizens' views of health equity in the emerging digital health landscape? Policy debates in the last few years have tended to focus on meaningful use and "patient engagement" and how to define these terms. The meanings of engagement and participation will emerge out of the multiple contexts in which people use the technologies, that is, social contexts, their understandings of their own bodies and disease, and the underlying economics of digital health, just to name a few dimensions. Andrew Barry's work on technological citizenship highlighted how citizens in the UK engaged with new sensor technologies that measured air pollution levels along freeways and in London. The reactions were often unexpected. Policymakers and technology developers often assume most "users" are relatively unsophisticated when it comes to technology. In this case, the sensors and real-time visualizations of pollution levels catalyzed vigorous public debate on the meaning of air pollution, questions of whose knowledge mattered in determining what level of a particular pollutant would constitute pollution. We should not be surprised if similar controversies arise in digital health. Putting technologies in the home means that homes will change in meaning. Different digital technologies will have differential impacts for patients with different diseases, different social contexts, and socioeconomic backgrounds. These differences will sometimes create tensions that digital healthcare professionals of tomorrow will have to work on with more engaged and sophisticated patients. Different will not necessarily imply negative but we will need to think more deeply about the risks and downsides or paint points of digital health in the coming years before we get taken in by too much hype about tricorders and bright shiny things. Patients and citizens will be the health professions' partners in this journey and we better get used to it. Welcome to digital health and the future.

Chapter 4
The Future of Aging and Digital Health

Jody Ranck

In the introduction to this book, we wrote about the fundamental shift in the demographic transition that has created a significant problem with a health sector that was designed for a very different epidemiological profile. In 1900, about the time that the foundations of our current health system were being created, the average life expectancy was around 47. Flash forward a little more than a century and life expectancies have now reached 78. As society ages, we are facing an expensive challenge when it comes to managing the health and wellness of a population that is living longer, and as we live longer, this often means managing more chronic diseases. The majority of one's health expenditures over the course of one's life are actually spent in the last two weeks of life—in the United States, we tend to die in hospitals receiving a great deal of expensive, high-tech care. In some countries, people tend to die at home. Anthropologist Sharon Kauffman wrote an award-winning book on aging and the end of life, *And a Time to Die: How American Hospitals Shape the End of Life*, where she explores the "gray zones" where patients have gone through intensive care treatments to prolong their lives and enter a place where they often have to face acute decisions that determine whether they live or die. They often cannot return home or return to a nursing home and are forced to enter more technologically focused institutions that can manage the level of care they require for their conditions. This is a situation that most of us are familiar with having watched a parent or grandparent in the final months of life. Witnessing the "gray zone" and the toll that this takes on individuals, families, and even healthcare providers has become an experience for many baby boomers that is helping to feed a different approach to aging.

J. Ranck (✉)
Health Bank, Ranck Consulting, Ram Group, Washington, DC, USA
e-mail: jody@ranckconsulting.com

© Springer International Publishing Switzerland 2016
J. Ranck (ed.), *Disruptive Cooperation in Digital Health*,
DOI 10.1007/978-3-319-40980-1_4

Baby boomers who came of age during the 1960s have been at the forefront of many of the major cultural shifts that have taken place over the last several decades. From the anti-war protests and civil rights struggles of the 1960s to a different approach toward experts and expertise, they are demanding new experiences and helping to redefine what aging means. This is the generation that is viewing retirement as an opportunity for a second career, if you are one of the one's fortunate enough to have invested and built up a nice retirement. For the lower income baby boomers, they may have different expectations about aging than their parents but all too often are struggling with a number of chronic diseases such as diabetes, obesity, asthma, congestive heart failure. It is the segment of the aging poor that have not had the access to preventive care and end up in acute centers of care more frequently that drive up healthcare expenditures. It is here where we will find many opportunities to use digital or wireless technologies to help reshape the experience of aging as well as provide both more cost-effective and more medically effective care in the coming years through sensors and telehealth technologies deployed at the home and even in the built environment around the city. *Yes, the city*. We should not lose sight of the broader context and a much broader agenda for technology and aging as we examine the new technologies that we will increasingly find useful in the home. Smart Cities may have plenty of room for innovations that make aging in the city a far more pleasant and productive experience. In fact, our views have been shifting for decades so that the image of the pensioner is shifting to a more active lifestyle.

Changing the experience of aging means facilitating the means to foster active, connected, and meaningful lives for seniors beyond just sensing health problems. Approximately one-third of Americans over 75 live alone and this frequently creates concerns for extended family members who want reassurance that their relative is doing well when there is no one else in the home to monitor or check in on a family member physically. In other contexts, the extended family makes this less of a problem, but we still need to think about how to enhance the experience of seniors as they age. This is creating a demand for telemonitoring products and services that can help caregivers and family members keep tabs on elderly friends and family from remote locations as well as wayfinding technologies. Sensors, the Internet of Things, and wearables may all have a significant role in the future of aging in place.

Boomer Expectations of Aging

The American Association of Retired Persons (AARP) regularly conducts studies on the needs and expectations of America's seniors and health is a major area of focus. Since the late 2000s, they have been conducting substantial research on aging, health, and aging in place through a program called Healthy@Home 2.0—the 2.0 implies connected and online. The assumption by many in public health over the years is that seniors do not use the internet. This has begun to change, and rather dramatically one might add. Simple tools such as email have been adopted by many of today's seniors, but baby boomers have been using their smartphones for the past several years as well. All of these technology practices are shaping the culture of aging. The result of some AARP surveys indicated that 9 out of 10 seniors now want to stay in their own homes as they age and up to 80 % of those over 65 are willing to adopt new technologies to age in their homes.[1] They are even willing to give up some of their privacy to do so.

The latest surveys from AARP also indicate that two-thirds of those over 65 currently use computers to communicate with family members and friends and the rate of change in knowledge of technologies since the survey was first done in 2007 is growing rapidly. While smartphones are not the norm across the spectrum of aging individuals over 65, access to cellphones and approximately 50 % of those interviewed have a strong interest in using their phone to access health information.[2] At the time of the 2010 survey, approximately one in ten was using their phone to track some form of health issue such as weight, blood sugar, or blood pressure, but many more were interested in adopting mobiles to do this in the future.

To get a grasp of the potential influence and market power of baby boomers, we will offer a few statistics:

• Nearly 78 million were born between 1946 and 1964
• One-third are online and they are one of the fastest growing demographics on some of the major social networking sites
• 68 % of the younger and 51 % of the older baby boomers use home broadband to go online
• 59 % have been caregivers to an aging relative for at least three years[3]

But beyond these statistics, there are expectations about lifestyles and health that boomers are making known to policymakers and companies. This is a generation that has been more engaged with politics, devours much more information, and is demanding a greater role in health and medical decisions. Many had (have) much more active lifestyles and came of age during the running and fitness booms that began in the 1970s. Their professional lives have seen the computer and smartphone go mainstream and they are often early adopters of new technologies.

While they may be adopters of technologies, they are also retiring in an age of rapid medical care inflation and general belt-tightening due to the financial crisis. Medicare typically only covers about 75 % of home care expenses and chronic diseases are driving growth in out-of-pocket medical care expenses for the aging.[4]

---

[1]http://blog.aarp.org/2012/07/09/aging-at-home-with-the-help-of-technology/.

[2]http://assets.aarp.org/rgcenter/general/health-caregiving-mobile-technology.pdf.

[3]Enterprise Forum Northwest, 2011, Boomers, Technology and Health: Consumers Taking Charge! http://www.mitwa.org/sites/default/files/files/MITEF%20NW%20Boomers%20Technology%20 and%20Health%20Report.pdf.

[4](ibid). Also see Chronic Diseases: The Power to Prevent. The Call to Control. National Center for Chronic Disease Prevention and Health Promotion, 2009.

When you combine this with the economic toll of caregiving that is estimated to cost individuals in aggregate about $350 billion annually, there may be some powerful financial drivers of adoption of technologies that can keep individuals out of the hospital and save money on overall health care spending at the household level. If these technologies can demonstrate their cost-effectiveness in the coming years, there will be many market opportunities for a spectrum of digital service providers from telecoms to cable. A report by the Urban Institute estimates that out-of-pocket expenses for health care will double from $2600 in 2010 to $6200 by 2040 with approximately 1 in 10 paying more than $14,000 in 2040.[5] What makes this worse is that median incomes will grow at a much slower rate than medical expenditure inflation and contribute to a growing financial burden for medical care in the coming decades. What this means is that about 60 % of the rising household income in this period will be consumed by out-of-pocket healthcare expenditures. Controlling these expenditures is likely going to become a major public policy issue as the financial pain of the healthcare sector bites into boomer retirement incomes.

Advancing the Meanings of Aging

The phenomenon of an aging society has spawned a great deal of research interest in how countries are going to manage the demographic transition and technology typically plays a major role. At MIT, they have created AgeLab as a research laboratory interested in driving innovation around aging services and technologies to achieve what they call "successful aging" for societies and individuals. Rather than launch into a catalog of all of the wireless technologies that can help the aging we think, it would be useful to explore some of the thinking around the meaning of aging and to explore some of the more thoughtful approaches that integrate technology into the aging experience in a way that is holistic combined with a bold vision for a technology architecture. Why does this matter? Well, quite simply, a catalog of gizmos and gadgets is not what we need and will not be successful at fostering a truly different experience of aging. Integrating tools in a seamless manner is going to be critical for success in this market niche. Doing that requires the ability to bring multiple stakeholders from the private sector and public sector and build the business practices, technology standards, and policy frameworks to enable widespread adoption and scaling up of efforts. As we move toward anytime/anyplace health at the intersection of aging and the home, for example, we need to step back from the mad race to bring one-off products to the market without regard to how a coherent, interoperable system can emerge. Data silos and complexities created by less than optimal interoperability will likely fail in

---

[5]http://www.urban.org/UploadedPDF/412026_health_care_costs.pdf.

this demographic. Within the formal healthcare sector, this is an extremely difficult challenge and one that we will be grappling with for years to come. While we may not be able to completely avoid the pitfalls and legacy systems of the formal healthcare sector, we need to bring together the stakeholders in the digital health and aging space to think about the big picture or we will likely face a lot of expensive failures that could undermine the promise of the technology down the road.

MIT's AgeLab has one of the more compelling visions for how to pull think about technology and aging that we think is worthy of exploration here. The AgeLab vision is based on three interrelated domains that form a system that supports successful aging. The domains are as follows:[6]

- **Infrastructure**: Places and things in the physical environment that impact aging such as the home, stores, hospitals, automobiles, community, airports, transportation systems, consumer electronics, medical devices, mobile phones, furniture. How do each of these interact and support independent living as well as "excite and delight" across the lifespan. Note the importance of emotional impact and not just a strict medical functionality as the privileged dimension of design.
- **Information**: How do older adults allocate attention, seek information and advice, and make sense of the issues that matter (finances, health and wellness, insurance, aging in place, long-term care, end of life planning). From this knowledge how can we design mobile communications to inform choices, reinforce positive behaviors, and get the right information to the right people at the right time when they need to make a choice?
- **Institutional Innovation**: How do business strategies and government policies affect older people and establish the context of society aging to become an opportunity rather than a burden? How can government services be redesigned to add value for older adults and can retirement be reconfigured to take into account the fact that many may pursue more active retirements than previous generations? Can aging be reconfigured as a source for economic opportunities?

These are useful questions to ask and can be used to help frame how we think about an ecosystem approach to aging in the context of digital health innovation. The director of the AgeLab wrote a policy brief several years ago, before the boom in mHealth, that most innovation in our increasingly tech-centric world is focused on innovation one-device-at-a-time. This device-oriented approach, while necessary from a company perspective, is not going to succeed in meeting the needs of an aging society and the *aspirations* of the boomer generation.[7] He utilizes a children's story, *The Little Mermaid*, to illustrate what is wrong with a device-oriented approach:

---

[6]http://agelab.mit.edu/successful-aging-complex-system.

[7]http://web.mit.edu/coughlin/Public/Publications/Coughlin-Lau%20Public%20Policy%20&%20
Aging%20Report%20Winter%202006.pdf.

Look at this stuff

Isn't it neat?

Wouldn't you think my collection's complete?

...Looking around here you think

Sure, she's got everything

I've got gadgets and gizmos a-plenty

I've got whozits and whatzits galore

You want thingamabobs?

I've got twenty! But who cares? No big deal

I want more

(Disney, 1989).

Our growing ecosystem of connected devices need to be connected to an underlying vision of connectedness that can be up to the task of making the experience of using the devices meaningful, in other words, not just another tracking device. Telemedicine, they argue, has been around in one form or another for forty years but has yet to receive widespread adoption. Personal Emergency Response Systems (PERS) have been available for falls and emergencies in the household for nearly three decades and are similar in price to a monthly cable bill but fewer than a million have actually used these systems. What explains the failure to realize widespread adoption in these cases? It is the **vision thing** according to Joseph Coughlin (Director, MIT AgeLab) and Jasmin Lau.

These authors call for a vision informed by a more creative use of our technological imaginations—the visions that created cathedrals rather than cottages in the twelfth and thirteenth centuries. This is a vision that goes beyond the pragmatic and the purely technocentric. They view the current approach to technology and aging as analogous to the age of the cottage builders that only exploit the most basic older adult needs. This is a technofunctionalist view that needs to be transformed into a more creative, aspirational paradigm that can truly improve the lives of older adults. To inform this transformational vision, they have modified Maslow's hierarchy of needs into an integrated framework that moves from a functionalist healthy aging paradigm to a quality of aging paradigm.

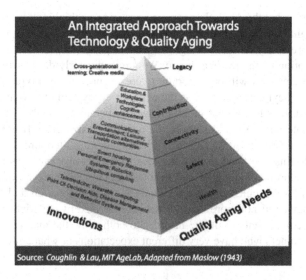

An Integrated Approach Towards Technology & Quality Aging

Source: Coughlin & Lau, MIT AgeLab, Adapted from Maslow (1943)

Health is focused on a construction of health and the body that views aging as synonymous with frailty and disability. Much akin to the manner in which many view wellness, their approach shifts to a vision that has positive connotations. We would argue that this problem plagues many medical and digital health devices that remind one of sickness and lack the aspirational elements that can engage individuals and communities. Technologies and services that want to make a difference with prevention will need to factor this into design and not remind one only of one's sickness or disease. Even when we are ill, or aging, we are more than sick and old. Coughlan and Lau remind us that many technologies are driven by government reimbursement policies that are slow to change and evolve with the speed of technological change.

Examples of how to make this shift include technologies that blend safety with social connectivity, for example. Staying connected while maintaining some autonomy, independence, and freedom to move around the home and the community are important and demand more than a device, but **collaboration between technologists and urban designers and transportation planners**. This is where some smart cities programs could make a difference if they move beyond a purely technocentric approach. We have seen the Wii appear in retirement homes and enhance the experience of living there by making life more fun and active. Technologies can be used to help build the confidence of older adults who may be losing some faculties while still have the ability to make a contribution to their communities and families. Being active in this manner, and sometimes with the assistance of cognition, enhancing technologies and brain gyms can play an important role in delaying decline in cognition. The authors also point out how many visual technologies are being used to enable the elderly to transmit their legacies to future generations and allow them to tell their stories to more people and in more creative ways. How often do we see storytelling as a feature in the digital health universe? Perhaps this needs to change.

In summary, what the AgeLab is espousing is systems thinking for aging technologies. For digital health to truly improve the experience of aging, we need to think about the entire ecosystem and design for a more people-centered experience even beyond the notion of the medical home. We are in the early days of implementing these technologies so it will be important to create space for this type of discussion that includes policymakers as well as the complex ecosystem of device manufacturers, broadband, healthcare, and mobile network operators to make the ubiquity of devices translate into a seamless, more life-affirming experience. If not, we should not expect the market to grow as much of the marketing literature indicates, quite frankly. To do this, we need to take the idea of cooperative business models seriously and develop methodologies and business models for this type of cooperative endeavor. This is difficult work and demands as much innovation and creativity as designing a device, if not more. Service design informed by experience design will be important components to utilize in order to both grow the market and meet the demands of boomers who have very different expectations of what aging means.

Aging in Place Technologies and the Market

Before we launch into our overview of wireless technologies for aging in place, it will be useful to introduce some trends in the market that will be shaping how the market matures in the coming years. Some of the challenges in the aging in technology market are linked to the overall financial crisis and the impact that the decline in incomes and assets has had since 2008. Some of the trends may have a rather ambiguous impact. For example, the number of nursing homes has actually decreased over the last decade with approximately 1000 folding between 2000 and 09.[8] Laurie Olov, an analyst with Aging in Place Technology Watch, notes also that the growth of non-profit and for-profit senior housing businesses and Assisted Living centers has stalled during the current recession. This has been a direct result of the housing crisis because many seniors who wanted to move into these facilities were unable to sell their homes and make the move financially feasible. Putting off transitions to these units has made the average age migrate to older adults in their mid-to late-1980s. Meanwhile, a large number of nursing homes surveyed indicated that they were not expecting to invest heavily in technologies. Therefore, technologies targeting the traditional set of facilities for aging may not see as bright a future as many would expect.

Where does this leave the home health market and various forms of the medical home? Orlov rightly points to the fact that home health care and personal aides have been one of the fastest growing sectors in the labor market in recent years, albeit these are very low-wage jobs.[9] Forecasts are projecting a 70 % growth in

[8]Magnolia Price survey, 2011.

[9]Orlov, Laurie, July 2012. The Future of Home Care Technology.

jobs in this category by 2020. Home care in these forecasts includes Companion Care (non-medical home care), home health care and geriatric care management. Orlov projects a $20 billion home healthcare technology market by 2020. While nursing home facilities have diminished over the past decade, the current reimbursement policy context that is focused on avoiding unnecessary rehospitalizations is going to become a big driver for adoption of remote patient monitoring devices that can facilitate self-care at arm's-length from the clinic. The challenge will come when we need to have home healthcare workers engaging with more sophisticated technologies and the additional training that will be required. Some in the industry have been talking about potential models from the "Geek Squads" from electronics retailers like Best Buy who can come to the home and help people set up their computers and home electronics systems. We can now also ask what Uber (yes, an overused analogy but sometimes useful for thinking beyond current constraints) for aging care would look like that could connect home health, technology, and seniors in a real-time, more productive manner. Health care is probably even more complex and home health workers are relatively low-wage, not highly educated positions.

On top of the auxiliary workers that may be needed to assist the elderly with both their health conditions and technologies deployed in the home, there is the challenge of getting the technology into the home and synchronizing the billing, installation, device makers, hospitals, primary and specialty care providers. This is an area that many of the broadband and telecommunications companies are increasingly lining up to fill in the gaps. A very fragmented system needs various types of integrators from data integrators to service integrators. Within the telecommunications arena, they are working to build frameworks that can be used for standards, benchmarks, and best practices in eHealth that can be shared across the industry and help catalyze growth by developing strategies that facilitate the integration function. Much of this work is directly relevant to aging in place. Our current paper-based system is a terrible way to go if you want the patient experience as they move from a hospital back to the home and are unfamiliar with some of these technologies. This type of system creates a burden for caregivers, patients and providers. But in most cases our current health IT architecture is not yet up to where we need it to be for making the experience along the continuum of care a patient-centric one, even though we as an industry tend to use this term a lot these days.

Some of the barriers to making an actual 'system' vs a cottage industry of fragmented service and product providers is the fact that we do not even have a shared vocabulary to talk about telehealth and telemedicine yet. Legal frameworks that address who is responsible if a power outage or equipment malfunction happens and jeopardizes a patient's life are just being developed now. This creates risks for companies wanting to offer these services because they must operate in a very litigious culture in the United States and elsewhere. On top of this, most hospitals have been struggling to implement EMRs for the past several years. This is a complicated technology implementation due to legacy systems and the number of information systems for laboratories, patient records, finance, and operations.

Now, when you add interoperability with a remote system in a patient home, the complexity goes up as well as the risks. As we will see in our chapter on the challenge of interoperability, improving interoperability can be a great thing for improving the care of the patient but with it comes the risk of privacy breaches. The more data flow, the greater the risk of data getting into the wrong hands. Health data are tightly regulated by HIPAA and the penalties are high for data breaches. This creates a risk averse culture in the health industry when it comes to adopting technology.

What all of this means is that cooperation is going to be one of the essential ingredients for future success when it comes to the medical home and aging technologies, just as it is for the rest of the eHealth ecosystem. The geography of health care is changing. In a digital health universe, your doctor's office becomes less important, although it would not fade away. The home begins to look and feel more like a clinic, to a small degree. Do people want this? How can the design of the tools make the perception of the medical home shift away from the clinical to more aspirational? The reason for low adoption may have many aspects that often go unnoticed in healthcare circles. The prevalence of digital health technologies in the home is actually quite low currently. Adoption of these requires those cathedral builders to come together and create an overall technology strategy that can bring the two orbits of the clinic and the home together—that is connectedness is more than a technological feat. Orlov's survey of home health care indicates that the use of some of the most popular digital health tools remains quite low, in the single digits in some cases such as blood pressure monitors that are used in about 14 % of the cases. Medication dispensers are very popular, but most of these are not connected.

One of the integrative functions that Orlov rather astutely observes will come into being in the next several years is the Home Care Information Network (HCIN). She defines the Network as:

> An interconnected set of information about care plan and status, independent of destination, that is about, for, and inclusive of the care recipient, care providers, and designated family members.[10]

The healthcare industry and policy landscape have been dominated by the development of the Health Information Exchange (HIE) as an integrator within the formal healthcare system, and Orlov is taking the idea into the realm of the more distributed healthcare system, a very important next step that will not be without challenges for integration into the formal clinical information architecture. This type of integrative innovation will be extremely valuable to bring together stakeholders along the aging tech and medical home ecosystem to put together the building blocks that can grow the ecosystem and market and make the experience of using these technologies a fundamentally different experience. The participatory EMR that brings together clinical data with the observations of daily life will

---

[10]Ibid. p. 9.

make this an invaluable foundation. Some of the layers of functionality and existing service and technology providers are presented below:

Technology	Purpose	Example/description
Care search tools	Locate agency or worker	Caring.com, CareZone, CareLinx
Family portal	Communicate care status to families	Ankota, CaringBridge
Environmental and health sensing	Monitor safety in the home	Philips Lifeline with Auto Alert, Healthsense
Social engagement	Monitor, communicate with care recipient	GrandCare, Independa
Telehealth/mHealth, PERS	Remote chronic disease monitoring, medical alarm	IdealLife, Care Innovations, LifeStation
Video	Nurse-telehealth patient	Caring Connections (Intel/ Pfizer)
Work management	Time, attendance, billing	Sandata, Stratis

Although digital health technologies for aging are still in their infancy, we have a number of examples that are early signals of where much of the field is going. These technologies tend to focus on chronic disease management, fall detection, cognitive enhancements, or tracking tools from those suffering from failing memory or dementia.

HealthPal, a product from MedApps, is one of the most popular chronic disease management tools. This is a device that can integrate data from a number of devices designed for the home including blood pressure monitors, pulse oximeters, and scales. The data are then integrated with the EMR or a PHR. MedApps is actually a good example of how a number of different tools and platforms in wireless health can be integrated for complex chronic disease management. The system uses cloud computing, a mobile device in the home integrated with a number of auxiliary applications (scales, bp cuffs, etc.) along with clinical records (EMR) and patient records. The schematic below provides an overview of the entire system.

Qualcomm has become a significant player in the home with the introduction of the 2Net Platform in 2011. This builds on the work of the Continua Health Alliance, a consortium of health technology and device companies that have collaborated to create standards for Bluetooth devices so that these can interoperate effectively. The 2Net Hub is one of the gateways that connects to the platform and is designed for all Bluetooth devices. The 2Net hub is a plug-and-play device that can integrate with virtually all existing medical devices and applications. The beauty of this device is that it stores the health data in the cloud where it can be accessed by a physician. The device can integrate data collected on your smartphone, and the data are secured and encrypted in compliance with Payment Card Industry standards (credit card). This is one of the first solutions to come to market that goes a long way in making the ecosystem of devices interoperable and easy to use, a very difficult challenge. Qualcomm is also opening up their system with an SDK so that developers can create new applications to interface with a 2Net API.

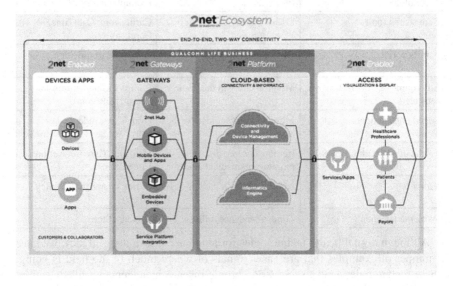

For patients with congestive heart failure, there are technologies that can monitor a number of vital signs and help patients manage their conditions remotely as well as have physician engagement. Coventis has developed the AVIVO Mobile Patient Management System that has a wearable monitor that patients wear on the chest. The monitor can communicate wirelessly with a physician platform that displays the data. The data include heart rate, fluid status, heart rate variability, respiratory rate, posture, activity, and ECGs. The platform does not require leads or wires nor does the user have to remove it when sleeping or in the shower.

Falls are a major cause of death and disability for the elderly and are expected to cause up to over $50 billion annually for the healthcare system by 2020.[11] Approximately 1 in 3 adults over 65 fall at least once per year and 20–30 % will suffer moderate to severe injuries from these falls. Approximately 662,000 are hospitalized for falls every year. Unfortunately, as many readers already know, falls can often lead to death due to traumatic brain injuries. As the elderly experience challenges with their gait or recover from strokes and other cognitive deficiencies, the risks of falls grow. This is a major reason why panic button technologies such as PERS were developed. Now with the next generation of wireless technologies, new approaches to fall management and detection are available. Often these technologies utilize the accelerometer in smartphones, or in wearable

---

[11]http://www.cdc.gov/homeandrecreationalsafety/falls/fallcost.html.

devices or in the home, some of the service providers can install sensors and video to detect movement, or lack of, and signal emergency services if necessary. More sophisticated monitors are in development that can actually predict the risk of falls in advance. Researchers at Texas Tech have developed a device that contains an accelerometer and gyroscope that can be attached to one's belt and record the patterns of the individual's gait and posture over time. They have developed algorithms that can detect shifts that are predictive of the risk of falling.[12] AT&T, as part of their mHealth work and efforts to connect household things and devices to the cloud, has developed "smart slippers" that contain pressure-sensitive sensors that monitor gait patterns, and when they detect a shift in the person's gait, an alert is sent to the doctor or caregiver for an intervention that may prevent falls.[13] For Android phone users, there is an app, iFall that uses the accelerometer and algorithms to detect falls.

Medications tend to enter our lives in greater abundance as we age. The average American is on about seven different prescription medications and many elderly are on even more. Adherence to the proper drug regimen is a challenge, particularly as the number of drugs increases or patients encounter failing cognitive capabilities. It is estimated that medication non-adherence results in 33–69 % of medication-related hospital admissions and these lapses are estimated to cost approximately $100 billion per year minimum and possibly up to $290 million according to the New England Healthcare Institute. Mobile phones have become useful for medication reminders and a number of applications, initially developed for low-income contexts such as South Africa for antiretroviral drug adherence programs, are now being used in the United States for aging populations. The Pill Phone is an application developed by Verizon and now used more widely is a medicine management software system that also has alerts.[14] Philips has developed a Medication Dispensing System that is about the size of a home expresso machine and dispenses medications on a set time schedule and alert caregivers when a dose is missed. Vitality Glowcaps are an example from the internet of things where sensors embedded in pill bottle caps have sensors that can detect the timing of doses as well as missed drugs and send SMS alerts as reminders to the patient. They can also be connected to one's social network to engage the network in peer support for taking the medication.

---

[12]http://www.medgadget.com/2012/08/new-wireless-sensor-can-predict-the-future-for-fall-risk-patients.html.

[13]http://mobihealthnews.com/5675/att-develops-smart-slippers-for-fall-prevention/.

[14]Many of the applications in this chapter are covered in more detail by the Center for Technology and Aging (2011). mHealth Technologies: Applications to Benefit Older Adults.

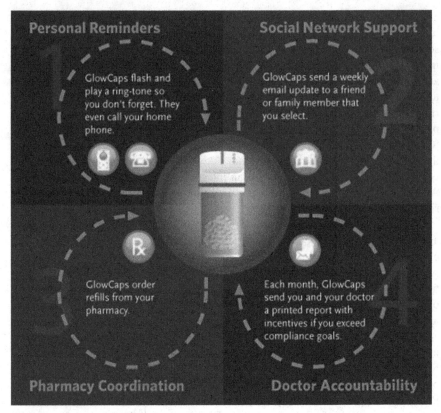

Vitality glow caps

Seniors with **dementia or Alzheimers** and related cognitive deficits are prone to wandering and caregivers often have to worry about the individual getting lost. Cellphones have become somewhat useful tools because they contain GPS, wifi, and other tracking technologies. The challenge has been to have technologies that work equally well in both indoor and outdoor settings. The Alzheimer's Association offers a technology called Comfort Zone that tracks patients and provides location data every 15–30 min and family members can use a number of different settings for alerts, tracking on a PC. There are other platforms such as EmFinders and EmSeeQ that are connected to law enforcement agencies. Google's Latitude application is also integrated with similar services.[15]

The US Veterans Administration has been an important supporter of telemental health services for aging veterans and veterans in general. More recent returnees from the Iraq and Afghanistan wars are now able to use mobile apps such as PTSD Coach to help them identify post-traumatic stress symptoms and seek help. Many veterans live in rural areas where access to mental health facilities is limited to

---

[15]Ibid.

telehealth applications that offer telecounseling sessions are available. Telehealth interventions could also be useful in transcending one of the barriers linked to stigma and mental health. If people can gain access to therapy in the privacy of the home, it could actually improve overall access to mental health.

Social supports and social networking are also available for aging adults. Throughout this book, we have discussed the growth and popularity of Health 2.0 sites and how these sites have begun to play a major role in the overall digital health landscape and provide excellent sources of peer support for managing chronic diseases, accessing information and providing a sense of community. This has not been lost on seniors who have become one of the fastest growing market segments in the social networking landscape. In the early days of the widespread adoption of social networking platforms, there were some senior-focused platforms such as Eons that have gone by the wayside as Facebook began to dominate the social networking landscape. And seniors are migrating to Facebook in impressive numbers and using it to stay in touch with family members. There are definitely socioeconomic divides in adoption rates and large numbers of low-income seniors who are not on the platform at all. Nevertheless, the medium could become a useful platform to address one of the barriers to adoption of aging technologies—lack of information.

In technology blogs, it is not uncommon to read about the role that robots are going to play in the medical home. Aging technology experts such as Laurie Orlov are quite skeptical about this happening anytime soon given the slow adoption of even basic technologies such as Skype in senior housing organizations. The prices are high and return on investment, or at least perception of ROI is too low at the moment. Robotic vacuum stories make good print in the tech blogosphere but are not generating a lot of excitement when it comes to the future of aging discussion. Future-focused studies often put these up front, we will refrain from this for the time being until we some convincing evidence that robotics will become more practical. This is not to say that they are not already an important feature of hospitals and other healthcare contexts. As researchers continue to work on interface design for robotics so that the human connection does not get lost, we may see inroads in this space, but there is still a great deal of debate over the fear of loss of the human touch.

Conclusion

To return to our discussion at the beginning of this chapter, we need to inject both pragmatic and visionary approaches to make the future of aging technology one capable of realizing the promise. We have offered a number of existing examples, but we need to generate a framework to guide policy and cooperation across the ecosystem to make all of these things work together and meet the needs of seniors who are more than sick and infirm individuals, but rather people who want to enjoy the twilight years and feel empowered to make more decisions. Baby boomers will probably want more than they can afford in our device-driven universe. But they will have to manage an ever wide set of options. When Jody worked for the Institute for the Future, some colleagues did some research on aging and came up with one useful framework for understanding how decisions will be made.

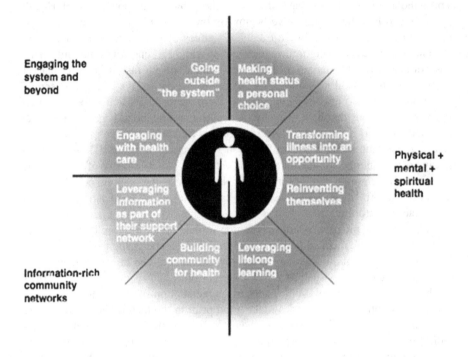

Boomer strategies for dealing with life transitions

This schema captures both the aspirational elements of aging with the diversity of tools and technologies that many baby boomers have become accustomed to given the general cultural shifts that they were part of since the 1960s. Design of aging technologies, to achieve high adoption rates, will need to transcend the medical device aesthetics and engage with the positive emotional elements of aging.

Later in this book, we will discuss the general challenge of interoperability that will be applicable to the future of aging technologies as well. The range of devices and telemedicine tools available to the elderly and the movement toward the medical home are slowly becoming a reality for seniors, but we are still in a market scenario where probably 10 % or less of those over 65 are using the technology. The future may happen faster if we take the advice of Joseph Coughlan and others who are espousing an approach that goes beyond the device and toward an aging systems framework. This could be helped by building bridges to stakeholders in city planning as well. Transportation networks, recreation, and the built environment need to be rethought in light of an aging society. The medical home cannot just be an island surrounded by the rough waters of non-interoperable, fragmented systems from the sickness economy framework. Smart cities have become a growing piece of business for companies such as IBM whose Smarter Planet initiative is helping city planners around the globe make better use of technologies and data. To date, these efforts have primarily been focused on economic development. The underlying theory of smart cities might want to consider integrating aging and health, but framed as opportunities for smart growth too. Too many ad hoc technology implementations in both aging and the city may only become barriers to the growth and innovation in this space in the future. Fortunately, we live in a time when many of the technology and communications companies are very interested in sitting at the table to discuss new ways of doing business and collaboratively developing benchmarks, standards, and best practices. It is time that we develop the innovative frameworks to think with that can come to the table and make sure that we have the institutional interoperability to make the cathedral vision of aging come into reality over the next decade. As in most of what we cover in this book, to implement the vision of a truly connected health framework will take planning and implementation cycles that go on for the next decade and longer. Even the way we evaluate the technologies will need to be rethought. Systems theory can inform evaluative efforts as well and this can only be accomplished through developing the leadership and frameworks for managing complex cooperative business models.

Chapter 5
From the Shrink in Your Pocket to the Quantified Self: Self-tracking and Self-care

Jody Ranck

Back in 2006, the editor of this volume (Jody Ranck) was co-directing the health practice at the Institute for the Future, a Silicon Valley think tank that studies technology trends, and we were holding one of our regular conferences on emerging technologies and business models in health care and trying to come up with some scenarios on where mobile health and personal heath technologies might lead in the coming years. Our conferences typically had a number of health executives, techies, and cutting edge thinkers from Silicon Valley. In one of our typical brainstorming sessions some of the personalities that tend to be on the cusp of emerging technology trends kept telling the audience that we needed to pay attention to some of the extreme athletes, typically cyclists and triathletes, who were tracking data on their workouts and diets. This was the future of health care some of them advised. Many in the audience shrugged. What does this have to do with health care? The explanation we heard was that more and more devices would be coming to market that enable us to track more and more vital signs and this would become mainstream in the health care sector within years.

The Quantified Self (QS) is described on the QS blog as "self knowledge through numbers" or "Quantified Self is a collaboration of users and tool makers who share an interest in self knowledge through self-tracking. We exchange information about our personal projects, the tools we use, tips we've gleaned, and lessons we've learned. We blog, meet face to face, and collaborate online."[1] If one

---

[1] http://quantifiedself.com/about/.

J. Ranck (✉)
Health Bank, Ranck Consulting, Ram Group, Washington, D.C., USA
e-mail: jody@ranckconsulting.com

© Springer International Publishing Switzerland 2016
J. Ranck (ed.), *Disruptive Cooperation in Digital Health*,
DOI 10.1007/978-3-319-40980-1_5

explores the QS blog and the forums on LinkedIn where practitioners meet and
share their self-tracking insights one is greeted with a very impressive range of
narratives and insights of individuals who have been tracking sleep, diet, food,
exercise, mood, supplements, sex, menstrual cycles, vital signs, and cognitive abilities—and sharing this data in many cases. From organized research efforts to
n-of-one accounts of self-experiments and studies, the movement is beginning to
make itself known in popular culture. Author Tim Ferriss and the popularity of his
books on work, diet, and exercise is one indication of the early mainstreaming of
self-tracking and "body hacking" as popular trends.

By 2007 Gary Wolf and Kevin Kelly, journalists and editor/founder of Wired
Magazine had coined the term Quantified Self and started writing a blog about
their own self-tracking efforts which soon led to a community of writers chroni-
cling their self-tracking efforts. Within a year or two meetups of the QS movement
began and we now see QS groups in over 50 cities worldwide. A number of
Silicon Valley venture capital firms have their eyes on innovative technologies and
companies that could push the trend farther into the mainstream and become the
next big thing in health care and health technology. In June 2015, Fitbit had an
IPO, one of the first for a wearable device or self-tracking maker and one that has
become synonymous with the QS movement. In 2010, Wolf wrote an important
essay on the QS in the New York Times Magazine entitled, "The Data-Driven
Life"[2] in which he highlighted the efforts of a number of individuals to solve specific behavioral or health problems through data collection about their lives and
conditions. He notes that data or numbers are changing the way government and
businesses work, so why not individuals:

> Numbers make problems less resonant emotionally but more tractable intellectually. In
> science, in business, and in the more reasonable sectors of government, numbers have
> won fair and square. (ibid)

He highlighted how this practice was actually quite widespread if we looked
across the Health 2.0 ecosystem, we could find large numbers of self-trackers. One
popular Health 2.0 site, MedHelp (http://www.medhelp.org/), had over 30,000 new
personal tracking experiments launched per month by 2010. What was driving this
was a number of important new trends. First, sensors got better—that is, cheaper and
smaller. Second, more people began carrying smartphones. Third, the social media
revolution had made sharing an important cultural phenomenon. Fourth, cloud computing was enabling more computing power to become even more ubiquitous.

One of the first areas to feel the impact of the QS movement is fitness. The
impact of these technologies was already playing out in the athletics arena as the
tools used to improve the performance of elite athletes had traditionally used video
and analysis of footage to improve technique. Now, with the growing availability
of sensors and accelerometers, we could use these at a much lower cost. The adoption of accelerometers by the auto industry for use in airbags had driven the price

---

[2]Gary Wolf, "The Data Driven Life", New York Times, April 28, 2010. http://www.nytimes.
com/2010/05/02/magazine/02self-measurement-t.html?pagewanted=all.

down such that they could be used in a wider number of devices. Combine sensors and accelerometers with data analytics and you have something quite valuable to the average person. Athletes had been self-trackers for years already but now the tools were becoming far more sophisticated, on one hand, and cheaper, on the other. You no longer needed to train with the US Olympic Team to have access to tools once used only by elite teams.

About this time, some of the tools for data analysis began to become cheaper and more user friendly as well. IBM released and open-source data visualization site called "Many Eyes" and for several years, we had a platform called Swivel that allowed anyone with a spreadsheet to upload their data and choose the data visualization format they preferred. This used to take a fair amount of training, typically a PhD or graduate degree in design to accomplish readily. The cloud, one of the fundamental technologies behind most social media sites that had begun to take off, was adding further momentum.

Wolf speculated that quantifying the self could offer advantages over traditional cognitive therapies in areas such as personal development because we now have the tools to understand many of the small things that could make a big difference in our well-being. Tracking tools enable us to conduct self-experiments in more empirical ways. Furthermore, even athletes are prone to bouts of self-deception— I'll round off my run or swim today to impress my training partners when they're not looking or fall off the diet for a few days. We may intentionally ignore what we don't want to face, but machines, he argues, don't have that option. *The cold, hard data could speak the truth*. This smacks of a hard-nosed empiricism that will undoubtedly rub many social scientists and psychologists who understand the interpretive dimensions of life rather differently. Improving the self is more than a data-driven empirical exercise. In reality, many of the practitioners of the QS movement don't inhabit a binary world of numbers versus context, but actively look for ways to integrate qualitative and quantitative approaches. There may be some shortcomings to neglecting the *Qualitative Self* that is more challenging to quantify. Nevertheless, the movement of self-trackers is taking off. There will likely be a point of reckoning where the limits of numbers become apparent, but there are substantial benefits to the way we think about medicine and norms. Wolf sees how the fetishization of numbers can sometimes lead medicine astray when he discusses an example of the use of "standards" for care and when you find out that your own situation does not fit the norm or the standard. Statistics deal in populations, physicians, and patients focus on individuals. Reality often lies in the movement back and forth between the two and quantitative methods will need to grasp this better in the age of population health management that concurs with patient-centric health and medicine. This is when the data one collects on oneself can potentially be life-saving or transformative in finding more personalized modes of care. This tension between the standard or evidence base and the individual, more personalized treatment is about to get interesting with the tools we have today and in the next few years. Digital health and analytics meet the reality of clinical workflows and patients' contextual lives and experience of disease. We won't win the battle by just throwing technology and numbers at physicians and patients. It is a far more complicated matter.

We're writing several years after the IFTF conference and Wolf's seminal piece in the *New York Times* and the self-tracking movement has moved beyond meetup groups and Silicon Valley. The Pew Internet and American Life Project conducted a survey during the summer of 2012 and found some interesting trends regarding the use of mobiles for health care issues[3]:

- 19 % of smartphone owners have downloaded a health app.
- Most of those downloading a health app are women who is better educated with a household income of $75,000 or over.
- One in three cellphone users have used their phone for health issues.
- 60 % of Americans track their weight, diet, or exercise routines.
- One-third of the survey respondents track a health indicator or symptom such as blood pressure, blood sugar, headaches, or sleep.
- One-third of caregivers track health issues of a loved one.
- 50 % of the trackers are tracking indicators in their heads and not on phones.
- Only one-fifth of the trackers use an app, cellphone, or online tool.

These data indicate both the promise and challenge of tracking applications in health care. On one hand, why isn't this number higher given the number of apps in the app store and the ubiquity of cellphones. Outreach and better apps that can sustain engagement of patients and those who are healthy in order to help them maintain their health status are needed. The science behind mobile apps needs to improve in order to justify the investment. We'll talk about gamification and gaming dynamics, often treated as the cure all for the challenge of patient engagement, but there is more to adoption than gamifying incentives. This also represents a potentially growing market opportunity for companies smart enough to marry the right behavioral change methodologies to mobile applications and creative uses of data for changing health outcomes. What the QS movement is creating is an important test bed for concepts and communities that may very likely hold one of the keys to the future of design and the entry of diverse other markets such as consumer electronics into the medical device and wireless health space.

The Quantified Self: From Silicon Valley Geeks to Mainstream Movement?

In the years since our Institute for the Future conference, this small band of trackers has emerged as a self-proclaimed 'movement'. They even have their own conferences well beyond the confines and 'bubble' of San Francisco with Wired Magazine even launching a new health platform around health data, tracking, and connected health technologies in early October 2012. Numerous Health 2.0 platforms emerged over the past several years that have leveraged the many-to-many

---

[3]http://pewinternet.org/Reports/2012/Mobile-Health.aspx.

sharing capabilities of Web 2.0 technologies to enable the scaling up of data sharing efforts of self-trackers to enable scientific research as an outcome of self-tracking practices. According to the Quantified Self blog's annual report, the number of Quantified Self groups grew by sixfold in 2011 alone.

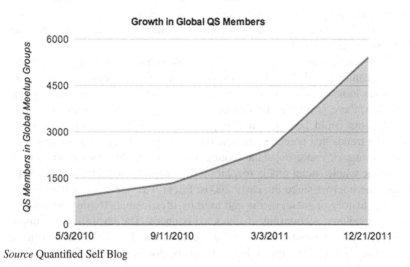

Source Quantified Self Blog

One needs to be careful in always assuming that big in Silicon Valley will become a global trend and all we need to do is wait a few years and early adopters will become the harbingers of mainstream trends. In this case, the term "Quantified Self" may end up not being the most scalable name for a trend and can actually be off-putting to many mainstream users of tracking devices, but there are a number of trends and figures within the movement that are worthwhile following to see where we may be headed in the self-tracking space. Employee wellness programs fueled by incentives in the Affordable Care Act (ACA) and employers' concerns for rising health care costs have been driving adoption rates of tracking devices for the past several years. There are now platforms such as Jiff that enable BYOD approaches so that employees can choose whatever tracking device they prefer.

Many readers may utilize popular fitness apps such as Runkeeper and MapMyFitness. Globally, these two apps alone have nearly 20 million users, many of them quite passionate and active users. In early 2015, the clothing manufacturer Under Armour acquired Endomondo and MyFitnessPal for over $500 million and acquired communities of over 120 million users worldwide. Popular dieting and food tracking apps such as Livestrong, LoseIt!, and the Weight Watchers apps also have impressive numbers of active users. Wearable technologies used for fitness and sports are exploding in popularity as well with devices such as FitBit, BodyMedia, Striiv's fitness monitors, Withings (body scale, smart watch, and blood pressure cuff), and Adidas Mi Coach, to name a few, have become very popular tracking devices that also connect to apps or platforms where users can share data and details on workouts with people in their social networks. At the end of European soccer games, we can see how far each athlete ran during the course of the match due to sensors in their athletic footwear. NFL spring training now sees rookies having their velocity and acceleration measured by wearables (wearable computing technologies) containing sensors that enabled coaching staff to follow their vitals remotely. In the next several years, the availability of these tools is likely to be given a boost by the entry of major consumer electronics companies into the broader eHealth space.

Fitness devices and the basic economics of health care are making mainstreaming of the Quantified Self look very attractive to a growing number of hardware manufacturers looking at the next big thing. With one-fifth of the economy going to health care, there is no wonder that devices equipped with sensors to monitor health indicators could be a possible opportunity. The QS movement taps into some broader trends that preceded the self-tracking for healthcare phenomenon.

Lifestreaming, or capturing data about one's everyday life, began to take off early on in the whole social media revolution that has shaped the contours of digital life and the internet since the early 2000s. Flickr was one of the early success stories in the history of social media and used by lifestreamers to provide a photographic documentary accounting of one's experiences. The term "lifestreaming" was coined by Yale computer scientists Eric Freeman and David Gelernter in the early 1990s to describe "a time ordered stream of documents that functions as a diary of your electronic life; every document you create and every document other people send you are stored in your lifestream. The tail of your stream contains documents from the past (starting with your electronic birth certificate). Moving away from the tail and toward the present, your stream contains more recent documents—papers in progress or new electronic mail; other documents (pictures, correspondence, bills, movies, voice mail, software) are stored in between. Moving beyond the present and into the future, the stream contains documents you will need: reminders, calendar items, and to-do lists."[4] If this looks familiar, it is because the concept became a central part of the Web as we know it today through the likes of Facebook, Myspace, and other social media sites.

Even prior to the lifestreaming movement, wearable computing pioneer Steve Mann (considered by many to be the first cyborg) had created a cyborg-like computer to capture all of his daily activities. Famously assaulted in the summer of 2012 in a Paris McDonald's by an employee of the fast-food chain who was annoyed by the wearable computing device Mann was porting to livestream, he has recently advanced the technology to the point where it now is attached to a brain–computer interface (BCI) and has now entered in the "mediated reality" space of thought-controlled computing.[5]

Lifestreaming meets data analytics in the area called "reality mining." Alex Pentland, a data scientist at MIT, has coined the term reality mining to capture the notion of the process of mining the "bread crumbs" of our digital lives. Email,

---

[4]https://en.wikipedia.org/wiki/Lifestreaming.

[5]His company Interaxon has a demo: http://interaxon.ca/.

phone calls, and social media "check-ins"—all of these leave a digital trace that may offer clues into how we are feeling on any given day. Given enough of these data points and mathematics, it is possible to create algorithms that are predictive of our moods and other aspects of our emotional and physical well-being. Most of the data points currently come from our mobile phones that have become passive sensors constantly collecting data that most of us are completely unaware of as we go about our daily activities. As we go through our daily lives, telecommunication companies can see our geographical location and when or for how long we call or use our smartphones. In aggregate, this data can be interpreted to reveal insights on our face-to-face interactions, social roles, and even the dynamics of social interactions at the level of an entire city. Albert-Laszlo Barabasi, founding director of the Center for Network Science at Northeastern University, has used data from mobile phones to develop predictive models that can predict a person's location, within a square mile, with up to 93 % accuracy.[6] The science of social network analysis that extends from human biology to social systems is going to become a powerful analytical tool when combined with the self-tracking data of many Quantified Self aficionados who can combine everything from genetic data to behavioral and environmental data to shed light on the complexity of the drivers for health outcomes. But reality mining has one important difference from your Facebook timeline—Facebook captures what you would like to share with others and reality mining comes closer to what you actually do.[7] Shades of big brother? Perhaps. There will likely be a great deal of discussion about privacy and the trade-offs as self-tracking technologies begin bleeding into the social tracking side as well. There are certainly trade-offs around individual privacy but if we can see benefits in smarter, healthier cities built upon these analytics, there may be ways forward on the policy front to engage individuals and communities. If data become merely the domain of private sector gain, we should expect organizations to demand more control over what data are collected by whom.

Some of the data points that can be collected include types of data from a person's voice that can indicate things such as depression or other dimensions of a person's emotional and physical status. Cogito Health (http://www.cogitocorp.com/) is a startup that is working in the area of detection of emotional status based on signals from an individual's voice. Their current applications include applications to analyze the voices of veterans returning from war for signs of PTSD. Another spin-off from MIT and Sandy Pentland's laboratory is Ginger.io whose focus has been on the development of diabetes applications that include machine learning algorithms that learn from one's cellphone usage patterns and will hopefully detect early signs of depression in a diabetic that can be an early indication of falling off the bandwagon for self-care. Once the early signs of depression are recognized an intervention can be prompted to provide the patient with social supports or other forms of support to keep that patient in compliance with their self-care regimen.

---

[6]Gregory Mone, 2011. This Man Could Rule the World. Popular Science, November 2011.

[7]Reinventing Society in the Wake of Big Data. A Conversation wth (Sandy) Pentland. The Edge. http://www.edge.org/conversation.php?cid=reinventing-society-in-the-wake-of-big-data. August 30, 2012 (accessed November 11, 2012).

Influential Data Scientist Dr. Stephen Wolfram added fuel to the QS movement after he released his personal data on his work behaviors and trends over the past twenty plus years in the spring of 2012. Wolfram, the founder of the computational software, Mathematica and the computational knowledge engine, Wolfram|Alpha, unveiled his "personal analytics" of his work life and productivity since 1989. The data included analytics of his email activity, keystrokes typed on his computer, daily number of meetings, phone calls, call duration, and pedometer activity. All of the data assembled and analyzed through his various products, created a picture of Wolfram's daily the day.[8]

What does this have to do with health? The act of lifestreaming and self-tracking is catching on and could become an important dimension of the personalized

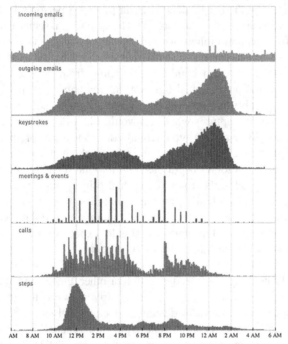

Wolfram's "Average Daily Rhythms"

or precision medicine of tomorrow.

We've already explored how expert patients or epatients are starting to drive change in health technology and a nascent movement in participatory health and medicine. An interesting health and medicine example that lines up nicely with Stephen Wolfram's self-tracking and personal data analytics is the experiments that Katie McCurdy, a designer suffering from myasthenia gravis, an autoimmune

---

[8]http://blog.stephenwolfram.com/2012/03/the-personal-analytics-of-my-life/.

disease. McCurdy has been taking prednisone for the past 20 years to suppress her immune system. Myasthenia gravis is a disease where one's antibodies attack the neurotransmitter receptors on muscles and cause fatigue, particularly with the muscles associated with the eyelids, facial expressions, chewing, swallowing, and even breathing. The disease can cause everything from impaired gait and difficulty breathing to changes in facial expressions. Prednisone, when taken for long periods can have numerous side effects including gastrointestinal problems. McCurdy had struggled with the side effects of Prednisone for years without much help in addressing these symptoms from a number of medical specialists. She eventually utilized her design skills to create a medical timeline that captured key data on the progression of her illness, side effects, medication usage, and dietary changes and created a "medical timeline" of her experience that could be shared with clinicians.

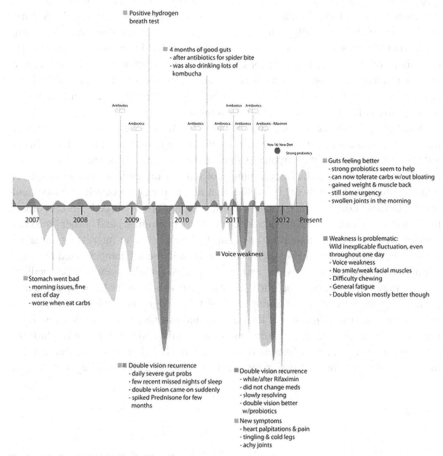

Katie McCurdy's Medical Timeline (http://sensical.wordpress.com/2012/01/03/medical-history-timeline-a-tool-for-doctor-visit-storytelling/)

The first time she took a copy of her medical timeline to the first clinical encounter with a new physician she reported that the data visualization gave her a stronger sense of empowerment when telling her medical narrative to the clinician. She felt that this form of self-tracking and data-driven story telling could prove very effective in jointly developing better treatment approaches.

The QS movement taps into another trend in the sciences that rises out of the nexus of the do-it-yourself, or DIY movement, and citizen science. Over the past few years, a movement around DIY genetics, often referred to as DIY bio or bio-punk, has been growing. The biohacking or biopunk movement includes both scientists and artists who are using the tools of genetics to raise awareness of how genetic information is being used while working to democratize access to the tools and technologies of biotech. Scientists and amateur or citizen scientists are hacking their way around IP-protected technologies to make more affordable means to do genetics outside of formal laboratories. Not without its critics and risks in areas such as biosecurity, biohackers have a number of new "hack spaces" to practice their craft including Genspace, a community laboratory in New York City, BioCurious in Silicon Valley. In these laboratories, hackers work on everything from microfluidics to diagnostics on open-source hardware sets. Some efforts even focus on collective research for cures via open communities and open-source approaches that focus on cures for breast cancer as we find in the work of the Pink Army Cooperative. Biopunk and DIY biohacking are helping to expand the realm of possibilities for the Quantified Self movement.

Another open-source science and technology effort is the open-source medical hardware community that builds on the open-source hardware of Arduino. This is a Radio Shack-like set of components that can be ordered online from outlets such as Amazon.com but also has a community of interest on medical Arduino applications.[9] LittleBits (littlebits.cc) is another that makes it easy to develop sensors and robots. In these communities, hackers are developing open-source heart rate monitors, pulse oximeters, biofeedback control technologies, and other medical devices. Why does this matter to the Quantified Self? It is an interesting signal of how medical knowledge and expertise are continually being democratized by communities of passionate activists and practitioners. While open-source medical devices may never become the norm, they are part of a broader hacking ethos that is changing the way we think about medical knowledge and devices. Hackers are also at work on filling in some of the gaps around interoperability of devices. Kyle Machulis, a self-proclaimed hacker, has set up a wiki and GitHub site (a platform for sharing open-source software) that is a forum for sharing open-source solutions or hacks that make it easier for users of devices to share and aggregate data

---

[9]Medicarduino.net.

across different fitness and tracking devices. His site, OpenYou.org has a number of hacks currently developed for FitBit, Nike Fuelband, and Emotive EEG devices.

Self-tracking and the Shrink in Your Pocket

The QS movement is not just about physical symptoms and fitness but also takes advantage of the mobile platform to track data that can be of use in the mental health arena. Mental health is probably one of the most neglected areas in our healthcare system. Stigma and excessive cultural baggage create tremendous barriers for many people to even considering accessing the mental health system, and often, it is a challenge to have health insurance that covers mental health services. Yet we know that mental health issues play a major role in everything from obesity to compliance with therapeutic regimens and all of these systemic failures have tremendous costs. There are some estimates that by 2030, mental health issues like depression could become some of the most costly in terms of overall economic burden on societies. While we don't expect mobile phones and telehealth to solve the overall challenge of mental health, we do see a lot of room for improvement and there are aspects of the QS movement that will be worth following in the coming years to see how they can provide inspiration for new ways of expanding access to mental health services as well as even improving our understandings of the connections between mental health and chronic diseases.

The failings of the mental health system are brought home when we look at the plight of returning veterans from wars in Iraq and Afghanistan and the challenges they face from war trauma. Mobiles and some of the tracking technologies we've been exploring here are quite relevant. The Veterans Administration has taken the lead with their work on the PTSD Coach app. One of the gaps in the system is the length of time it takes from when a veteran feels that he or she needs mental health assistance and the time they actually receive it. PTSD Coach was developed to help veterans to recognize the signs of distress, access strategies to manage their symptoms, and find the closest mental health providers. The early trials of the app were conducted in collaboration with the Open mHealth Project, an open-source architecture project that we explore elsewhere in this book that focuses on creating the backend architecture so that apps and data collection efforts can be integrated and interoperable. The VA and Open mHealth Project have also collaborated to develop PTSD Explorer that offers data visualization capabilities for clinicians and patients to have better ways of seeing what is going on with symptoms and care and eventually improve outcomes. This example illustrates some of the potential for mobiles for more acute mental health issues.

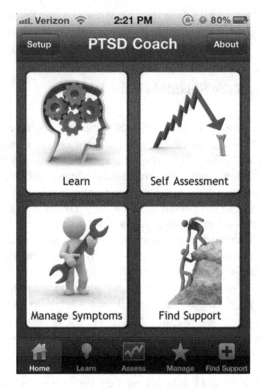

One of the most popular tracking items for QS followers is mood and emotional status. From athletes to those suffering from chronic diseases, mood can be an important factor in the overall equation determining outcomes. A number of popular mood tracking apps exist on the market and include Mood Panda, Buddy, Moody Me, My Mood Tracker, Mobiliyze, Viary.Se, and iCouchCBT. Many of these apps are simple tracking devices that act as "smart diaries" recording one's general emotional status alongside other indicators such as exercise, diet, and sleep so that the user can see how other factors may correlate with mood or emotional status. Viary is one of the first mental health applications to have undergone a clinical trial for use in treating depression.[10] In the first trial of this nature, over 80 subjects participated for over 8 weeks in a trial to assess the role of the Viary app in treating depression. The Viary app was compared to a mindfulness app not specifically designed for depression. Viary offers coaching and suggestions for activities and behaviors that can help a depressed person self-manage depressive episodes. At the end of the study, over 73 % of the users of the Viary app were no longer reporting the original depressive symptoms.[11] The makers of Viary are tar-

---

[10]Kien Hoa Ly et al. 2012, 13:62, *Trials*, Behavioral activation-based guided self-help treatment administered through a smartphone application: study protocol for a randomized control trial. http://www.trialsjournal.com/content/pdf/1745-6215-13-62.pdf.

[11]http://venturebeat.com/2012/05/30/app-cure-depression/.

geting the app for therapists, human resource managers, and lifestyle coaches because it enables the collection of data that can help both therapist and client monitor progress and behavior in between visits.

Many self-trackers are quite passionate about exploring the factors that can impact their moods. Mobiliyze resembles some of the reality mining apps mentioned earlier that track your location, level of physical activity and social interactions to detect whether the user could be feeling isolated. Billed as a "therapist in your pocket," the app will then send the user advice on activities that could help improve one's mood. Mood Panda is a similar app popular among QS practitioners that is a mood journal or diary and offers data visualization tools to display your aggregate data. It even allows one to compare one's mood with others, a popular activity in some quarters of the QS movement where data sharing is a central element of the self-tracking experience.

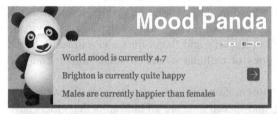

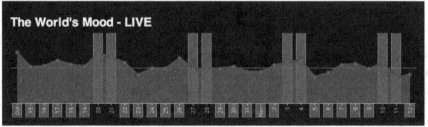

The app is marketed beyond those diagnosed with clinical mental health issues but for the general public merely interested in tracking moods and gaining insights into what potential influencing factors could be.

The valuable feature with the mood trackers is the ability to track changes in moods throughout the day and the contexts in which these moods change. The hardcore practitioners of the movement also have at their disposal a number of other tracking devices that can measure everything from sleep to food and alcohol consumption to build a rather comprehensive "health graph." Zeo was a device company that focused on sleep. Users wear a headband at night that can track your deep and REM sleep quantitatively. The MyZeo app then offers an analysis of your sleep with suggestions on how to improve your sleep outcomes. The company offered a great deal of suggestions and insights about the science of sleep and how to "hack one's sleep," in other words, they offered ideas for self-experiments that one can do in conjunction with using their device that could help you to improve the quality and quantity of sleep. One interesting note is that Zeo had become the largest database on sleep data in the world from all of the user data they have collected. Given the role that sleep plays in overall health outcomes, Zeo could have potentially been sitting on a major data goldmine in the coming years if they could have combined other streams of data with their sleep data. But Zeo became a case study of the difficulty in building viable business models in this space when it went out of business in 2013. Newer companies such as the Finnish-based Beddit have learned from the mistakes of Zeo and offering new sleep moni-toring technologies that are not worn on the body and less intrusive to sleep while offering more accurate monitoring of sleep without being medical diagnostic-level quality. Professional sports teams such as the Los Angeles Lakers are using the devices to avoid over-training and burnout of their athletes.

If you're having trouble sleeping perhaps, it is too much coffee late in the day. Well, there's an app for that too. Caffeine Tracker developed by scientists at Penn State University helps you optimize caffeine intake to stay alert when you need to and not to overdo it when you need to sleep. Based on peer-reviewed research studies on the metabolic rates for caffeine, the app allows the user to input the amount of caffeine consumed in milligrams and then offers a visualization of the metabolic rate or pharmacokinetics of caffeine based on some norms from the research literature.

The technology for monitoring emotions is improving as well. Galvanic skin response, respiration, heart rate, and speech tone are all indicators that QSers have begun monitoring to enhance their quantitative repertoire.[12] This area is now head-ing into the area of cognitive tracking. An interesting platform that emerged is the Quantified Mind (http://www.quantified-mind.com/) that helps you and a growing community of trackers explore what factors influence your mental performance. These "mind hackers" can join a number of experiments that explore everything from how eating breakfast impacts performance to the role of sex, coffee, or medi-tation on your mental acuity. And before we forget, there are trackers to monitor your sex life as well! The Quantified Mind has developed a number of tests to help one analyze and quantify various aspects of one's cognitive abilities including reaction time, verbal learning, context switching, short-term memory, visual per-ception, motor skills, and high-level processing abilities.[13] One can enter a number of academic studies sponsored on the site by registering and taking a given test. However, the selling point of the Quantified Mind is that they offer a platform that will actually let one empirically test the impact of different behaviors on cognitive outcomes through the use of psychometrics.

Lumosity (http://www.lumosity.com/) is similar to the Quantified Mind but it ascribes to the "brain hacking" point of view by offering tools and games that use research from the areas of neuroplasticity and fluid intelligence to improve your memory, problem-solving ability, and other cognitive functions.[14] Quite a few QS

---

[12]http://quantifiedself.com/2012/11/matt-dobson-on-quantifying-emotions/.

[13]http://www.quantified-mind.com/science.

[14]http://blogs.hbr.org/cs/2012/10/four_new_tools_for_brain_worko.html.

thought leaders do a bit of experimentation in this space and frequently present at the meetups. One notable example is Tim Lundeen who did a simple experiment on cognitive ability to see whether DHA (from fish oil) could improve his ability to do math problems over time. He gradually increased the dosage of DHA over 130 days. By day 80, he reached double his normal dosage and the time required to complete a math problem decreased.[15]

Food is an another important driver of health outcomes that is a natural area for QS practitioners to direct their attention. Several mainstream applications such as LoseIt! and Livestrong have become popular with the public at large as apps that can help you manage your diet and eating behaviors as well as fitness. Apps like these, along with the Weight Watchers mobile app, have extensive databases that allow users to input their meals and receive data on the number of calories as well as a brief snapshot of the nutritional content of the meal. One of the challenges with these types of apps is that the data input is only as accurate as the user input. Estimating the serving size of an average dish is going to carry a range of error with it unless you're eating at home and have a set of scales or the eating establishment has a precise measure on the package. Humans are notoriously bad at tracking their own meals in self-reported studies. This has been one of the big problems with a very popular eating and diet app created by Massive Health and later acquired by Jawbone. The Eatery was the first app released by Massive Health, who received over $10 million in venture funding. The app allowed the user to take a photograph of a meal, rate it in terms of how healthy it is, and then post the photograph on the app. Other users of the app then get to "crowdsource" their own rating of the relative healthiness of the meal. The problem with this app is the validity and reliability of data. As any health professional or QS practitioner knows, context matters. If I have a food allergy that meal that looks healthy could be toxic but the crowd might rate it as extremely healthy. Massive Health was known for their beautiful infographics but many in the healthcare world question the usefulness of the app as it now stands. And this is one of the questions that is going to continually arise in the coming years is when to jump on the bandwagon of an edgy trend like crowdsourcing and when is it actually producing useful new knowledge. Massive Health was eventually acquired by Jawbone to join the team building the Jawbone UP software and integration tools for users to track multiple biometric indicators and the company now competes head on with Fitbit for the lead in the domination of the tracking market.

A big part of the QS conferences and meetups is the sharing of insights and data. One can visit the LinkedIn group for the Quantified Self and at any given time come across surveys asking participants to share their own experiences and insights on everything from nutritional supplement usage to the calibration and accuracy of fitness devices. It is quite surprising sometimes just how passionate the QS community is. At one point, there was a very interesting discussion taking place over which fitness trackers provide the most accurate readings of exercise

---

[15]http://hplusmagazine.com/2010/02/08/self-tracking-quantified-life-worth-living.

and distance completed. It is impressive to see actually how many contributors to the discussion had already been using multiple devices at a time and had uncovered rather large discrepancies between devices such as FitBit, Nike Fuel+, Striiv, and other devices. Rachel Kalmar is a data scientist at Misfit Wearables who wears over 20 wearable tracking devices per day as an experiment to see how devices differ, the usability of platforms and any other insights she can gather from the data. A major interest of hers is how to break the devices out of the data silos so that more can be done with the data and ultimately lead to better applications and data services that render the devices more useful.[16] The future of many of these devices lies in the ways they will communicate with one another and tack back and forth between the body and contexts as well as other people.

Health 2.0 Meets the Quantified Self

Earlier, we mentioned online communities such as MedHelp that have users in the tens of thousands and many are engaged in some form of self-tracking and sharing of data. In the first few years of the QS movement, a number of these platforms became important catalysts for scaling up efforts and actually changing the way research was being conducted. One of the first was the platform called "CureTogether." CureTogether was launched in 2008 by Alexandra Carmichael, who had been suffering from a chronic pain issue that defied adequate diagnosis from mainstream medical practitioners. She founded CureTogether with her partners to offer a community for trackers to explore their conditions collectively. By the summer of 2012, the online personal genomics platform 23andMe had acquired CureTogether in order to scale up research efforts that bridged genomic data with phenotype data that had been collected by over 25,000 member of CureTogether's community. By 2012, CureTogether's platform had over 300 medical conditions that they were collectively sharing data and researching. The CureTogether community had reached a level of proficiency in tracking and research that a number of major academic and pharmaceutical company collaborations were under way.

What accounted for the popularity and research potential of CureTogether? The story of the founder is quite illustrative in this regard. Trained as a molecular biologist, Alexandra Carmichael had witnessed the challenge of chronic pain both personally and through a parent.[17] Her mother had experienced migraines throughout

---

[16]http://www.fastcolabs.com/3036433/elasticity/misfit-engineer-rachel-kalmar-wants-you-to-be-an-intelligent-node.

[17]http://www.thefifthconference.com/topic/health/how-curetogether-enables-patients-drive-medical-innovation.

Carmichael's childhood and she had herself experienced vulvodyna, chronic pain of the vulva. Physicians had failed to find a causal mechanism for her vulvodyna so she commenced upon her own research to figure out what could be causing the pain. She found disease support groups but felt that what was lacking was quantitative, evidence-based knowledge. Being in the midst of Silicon Valley during the social media revolution that was well underway, she launched CureTogether to help conduct research on vulvodyna, migraines, and endometriosis. As the community grew, so did the number of conditions and this actually contribute to the value of the platform. The healthcare system is not that good at dealing with comorbidities. CureTogether's research that is patient and experience-driven developed a strong emphasis on these comorbidities. It also added a bit of transparency to the research and medical practice space by allowing patients to plot data around treatments and outcomes. What came out of this frequently was the fact that the most popular treatments were often not the best.

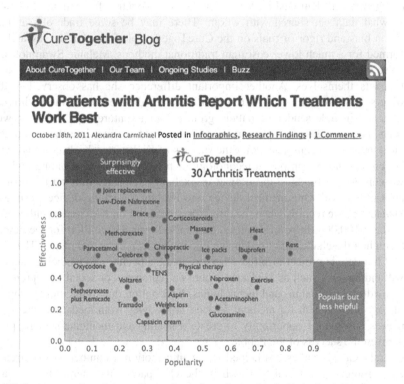

While not conforming to the strict rules of standard clinical trials, the surveys and research conducted by CureTogether are valuable in that they are a good indicator of the actual patient population for a typical disorder. Companies and academic researchers find these more participatory trials useful.

CureTogether has some additional unique aspects from the sheer volume of data collected by their members. With well over a million data points, the site has become the largest comparative effectiveness database accessible to patients in the world.[18] The acquisition by 23andMe opens up many new possibilities that can link health outcomes to not only genetic data, but behavioral and environmental data for more realistic models that come closer to real-world drivers of health outcomes. Big data analytics are making it cheaper to do this kind of research and integrate a vastly wider set of sensor data into the analytics. From the data that CureTogether already collects they have the capacity to build data visualizations and infographics that could shed light on the preferred methods that patients have for making sense of data. Sense-making and patient engagement are going to be critical to the success of wired technologies, and sustaining engagement has been a difficult challenge across the field. Mere participation in a project that is larger than oneself or one's tracking device can be a life-changing experience if you've been suffering in isolation with a difficult chronic condition or rare disease.

When one mentions patient-driven research, one of the first things that comes out of health researchers mouths is the issue of privacy. Platforms such as CureTogether and PatientsLikeMe do enable strict control for patients to determine what data get shared with whom. There may be some trade-offs around selection bias and rigor of trials on the CureTogether platform, but the research is performed for a much lower cost than traditional methods, Melanie Swan notes.[19] She also notes that the rewards of the research accrue more directly to the research participants themselves. Another important difference she has observed is the funding sources for this type of research are often different from the traditional sources and include academia, patient groups, social venture capital, and crowdfunding. The crowdfunding phenomenon is beginning to enter into the health and medical arenas in recent years after the success of Kickstarter. Kickstarter is a site where entrepreneurs can post a technology or project that needs funding and the crowd can donate funds to the project in exchange for early dibs on the project when it is released. One medical device, the Pebble, a tracking device worn as a wristwatch, broke records when the developers posted it on Kickstarter with a goal of raising $100,000. In several weeks, they raised over $10 million for the device and then had the challenge of producing enough to keep up with demand. The success of the Pebble project inspired others to create a health- and medicine-specific crowdfunding sites such as Medstartr where entrepreneurs or social entrepreneurs can crowdfund campaigns and technologies. Kickstarter, due to the more complex regulatory environment for medical devices, shies away from medical devices, so there was an obvious opportunity to create a health- and medicine-specific platform given the success of the Pebble.

Overall, CureTogether has helped to set into motion a number of new trends that are going to be useful to watch in the QS space. First, some diseases are found in such small numbers that the market has little interest in pursuing

---

[18]http://blog.makezine.com/2010/09/17/curetogether-crowdsourced-health/.

[19]Melanie Swan (2012). Crowdsourced Health Research Studies: An Important Emerging Complement to Clinical Trials in the Public Health Research Ecosystem. J Med Internet Res 14(2):e46.

cures. Otherwise known as the orphan drug problem, there are policy measures around orphan drugs that can help create funding incentives to get companies to do research in these areas but platforms like CureTogether offer an alternative approach that also offers sufferers of rare disorders to become part of a community that is actively engaged in self-care and research. This can help overcome some of the challenges such as isolation and lack of information about their conditions. Another feature is that CureTogether actively works on improving the quality of health information that people have access to. This is one of the big concerns around Health 2.0 and the Web for doctors. There is a lot of unverified, inaccurate health information on the Web. The larger Health 2.0 sites have communities that can act as filters and help sort dis/misinformation from the information that is relevant and medically verified. Of course, there will be gray areas where the medical literature does not have a firm answer, but even these areas can become focal points for the communities to focus on research, often in collaboration with clinical researchers to fill in the gaps faster. As mentioned earlier, some of the disease groups have actually conducted research that has proven that standard therapies used for ALS, such as lithium, were not as medically effective as health professionals had thought. This came about through patients sharing data and analyzing health outcomes.

As the citizen science and QS trends take hold one of the challenges has been the aggregation of data and making is easier to make sense of all of the data collected. We'll talk more about big data and data analytics in the overall wireless health space in our chapter on data, but the experience of using these devices could be made more patient-centric if we moved beyond the data silos that many devices create. If you used a Nike Fuelband, you might have found that it is a challenge to integrate the data with data collected from another device. Many companies are using APIs to integrate data from different devices and then build apps that allow you to create charts and other data visualizations. Withings, glucose monitors, Runkeeper, etc. all have APIs and we are beginning to see a new generation of API-driven innovation through the aggregation of data that can then analyze multiple data streams. Once one has access to the analytics tools running on top of a data warehouse or application then the possibility for coaching engines and approaches to behavioral modification can become more personalized and even delivered in real time during a workout or based on a prompt from a given data point, an alert for getting up and moving, for example.

Gamification of the Quantified Self and Crowdsourcing

Sustaining engagement with tracking often takes incentives and social community to keep people engaged with tracking for longer periods of time. Crowdsourcing of scientific research can also leverage incentives and games to increase data collection and even optimize problem solving on various platforms. In our introduction, we introduced the bioinformatics game Foldit that used crowdsourcing and game dynamics to engage laypersons in helping to unravel the folding dynamics of proteins necessary for new HIV therapeutics. Over the past year, a number of new startups have entered the market at the nexus of the QS movement and data visualization. TicTrac is a platform that is targeting the tracking market segment and makes it easy for self-trackers to upload data and generate data visualizations of their data. We should expect a convergence before long where data visualization and information design come together with mobiles, crowdsourcing and gaming dynamics not only to make tracking fun but also to enhance the esthetics and ability to make sense of the growing amount of data we'll be collecting.

Fitness has already entered the gamification of tracking and motivational behavior space with examples like Striiv, the pedometer/fitness tracking company. They've developed a small digital pedometer that tracks your steps and gives badges to users for achieving a goal for distances traversed. This is not that remarkable in itself until they offer the opportunity to donate "steps" to one's favorite charities like GlobalGiving.org. A play on this has been to have users of fitness devices choose the causes they actually despise, for example, a Democrat could choose a Republican cause, and wager a set amount of funds per month or week that will go the chosen cause if one fails to comply with a fitness or diet regimen. GymPact uses this type of incentive scheme to ensure compliance with a weekly fitness regimen.

We can see how the QS trend is beginning to feed into a number of the major themes of this book. From mobile devices to big data and gaming, the QS has become an important practice area to follow if you want to gain insights into the future of health and medicine. The infographic below highlights the convergence of these trends.

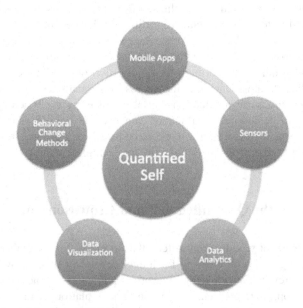

The Five Pillars of the Quantified Self

As the field continues to grow, we will likely see a shift in language from the geek terminology of the "Quantified Self" to more mainstream self-tracking terminology that also reflects the fact that self-tracking has a very long history that goes back many years. In 2014, we also saw many of the large technology platform players such as Google, Apple, Samsung, and WebMD enter the fray. Everyone appears to agree that health data could become big business in the coming years. This raises questions of who benefits, what is the business model and how the ecosystem of digital health devices itself may change as the adoption rates scale.

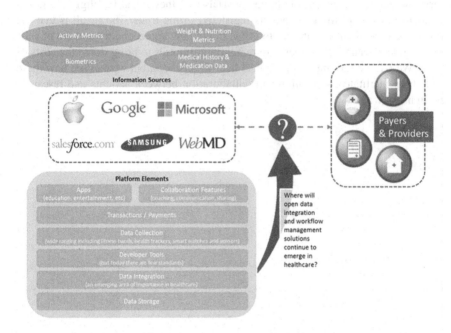

Betting on 'Switzerland' in Connected Health. *Source* Triple Tree

The boundaries between fitness and health care will blur in some respects. Since the passing of the Affordable Care Act and the rise of value-based care emphasize outcomes, lower costs, and population health improvements, we have seen the traditional way of thinking about health care as divided into payers, providers, and patients begin to shift. Providers are acting more like payers with a focus on lower cost care and outcomes; payers are buying providers. The front door of the health care may someday not be the front door of the clinic but one's house, the street or on your wrist or elsewhere on the body. As the QS phenomenon goes mainstream, whether self-tracking becomes focus actually misses the point. The rise of wearables, telehealth, and data analytics will enable new business models for real-time, real-world, anytime, and anyplace healthcare delivery models. While the idea that doctors will be replaced by computers seems a bit farfetched, the way that doctors and systems deliver care at arm's length is becoming a reality. There will be many planks built into the platforms illustrated above that provide new healthcare services and will aim to do a better job of providing more patient-centric care. This "platformification" of health care is already visible in the early days of some of the first steps that platforms such as Apple have initiated. In early 2015, Apple released Research Kit, an app that collects data from apps on your phone and can share this data with clinical researchers. In the first two days of the app's existence, more people enrolled in clinical research studies than would have been enrolled in one year through 50 different medical centers! This addresses one of the major obstacles for clinical research and clinical trials where very few people are aware of studies or trials that they could be eligible for, and it has been difficult to keep patients registered in the trials. The result is that the cost of new medicines continues to grow. In the new app economy and era of self-tracking devices and apps, there are many opportunities to bring down the costs of trials. We will be turning to this subject later in this book but we can see how these tools help facilitate cooperation and collaboration between patients and researchers in novel ways.

Chapter 6
The Data Revolution: Networks, Platforms, and the Data Sciences in Health

Jody Ranck

Why Health care Is and Isn't a Data-Driven Science?

The digital health (r)evolution may ultimately succeed or fail based on how we use data to change our behaviors, policies and organizations over the coming years. In order to see why this is so we will examine some of the health data challenges that our system has been struggling with over the past decade or so and why these problems will only grow unless the healthcare system becomes a more data-driven system as a whole. Medicine at the bedside is an empirical, data-driven science but also an art based on a subjective evaluation of the patient's social context, behavior and psychology. While the evidence base for medicine is based on the averages of large studies or trials, physicians treat the n of 1, meaning an individual. One's doctor is reading your symptoms as a number of data points based on your vital signs, laboratory diagnostics, and so on but also must evaluate these numbers in light of your own particular historical medical record and context. The challenge is that we find dramatic differences in how medicine is practiced and unfortunately there are large variations in how physicians treat a wide number of diseases even when there is an evidence base to guide and standardize treatments. When we hear that artificial intelligence and big data will replace doctors someday, we need to pause for a reality check in light of these aspects above.

In this chapter we will look at the research at Dartmouth Medical School that has documented treatment variations across the country over the years and explore the tension that occurs between globalized norms and the art of medicine at the bedside. On the surface these may appear to be at odds, but there are technological and

J. Ranck (✉)
Health Bank, Ranck Consulting, Ram Group, Washington DC, USA
e-mail: jody@ranckconsulting.com

© Springer International Publishing Switzerland 2016   103
J. Ranck (ed.), *Disruptive Cooperation in Digital Health*,
DOI 10.1007/978-3-319-40980-1_6

scientific developments that may help us to remedy some of the tension as the data sciences help to create a more personalized form of medicine while also making healthier populations in the coming years. This tension between personalization of therapy at the genetic level and the need to address public health issues is a very important one. This is where the data you collect on your mobile phone can be married with large data sets to help customize your treatment while simultaneously contributing to research that can help us find better treatments, risk models, and public health interventions customized for the type of neighborhood where one lives.

From a broader health system perspective we can use data analytics to help address inefficiencies. Our healthcare system is notoriously inefficient as the Institute of Medicine and many other studies have shown. Population Health Management has become the mantra as value-based care begins to grow in the US healthcare system. Analytics tools will be used to address many of the inefficiencies and gaps in the system through the following types of analytics tools:

- Risk stratification and predictive analytics for identifying high-risk patients and customizing treatment plans and identifying the most important care gaps
- Remote monitoring to gauge compliance and early warning systems when patients are at risk of declines in health status or non-compliance
- Community-level data for building effective collaborations between the clinic and the community (e.g., GIS, prevalence data, access to care data, hotspots of high utilizers of the system).

Obtaining real-time data on health system utilization and financials will be central to reforming the healthcare system. Many would be surprised to know that the average CFO of most hospitals has little understanding of the underlying costs of heart surgery, for example. Data services will offer one important avenue to realize efficiency gains and understanding the true costs of care. Unpacking the cost structure of care can also shed light on where processes can be improved and where technologies could be used to improve efficiencies in care and the allocation of resources. Using data in novel ways to improve clinical trials, to identify high-risk individuals and communities, and better targeting and coordination of care alone can help make dramatic improvements in the overall health system. But lack of interoperability and data silos are major challenges, particularly for Accountable Care Organizations (ACOs) needing real-time data, and many of the business offerings in the data analytics space are providing cloud-based solutions and using open APIs to break these silos and integrate diverse data streams.

There is another important driver that will make data analytics and big data even more invaluable and that is the gradual shift to a more prevention-focused or value-driven healthcare system. An important part of the Affordable Care Act is the creation of ACOs that function as an incentive for healthcare providers to coordinate care and improve the quality of care in the process. The traditional fee-for-service system that has dominated most US health care outside of the Kaiser Permanente's and Group Health Cooperatives (Puget Sound) has been one that rewarded doctors for the more tests, procedures, referrals, etc. that they prescribed. This has been one of the primary drivers of escalating healthcare costs. ACOs address this problem by paying a group of providers a set amount for a patient population, otherwise known as a bundled payment. If hospitals see preventable readmissions after hospital stays they will not be reimbursed, and in fact, could be penalized. This shifts the incentives toward a more prevention-focused mind-set. Prevention means knowing who is at greatest risk for high-cost procedures and readmissions and intervening proactively to prevent adverse outcomes and hospitalizations. Providers will increasingly administer Health Risk Assessments (HRAs) to patients who can then be stratified by risk and directed into a care plan and care management team who will collaborate using a variety of platforms that enable sharing of data and tools that enable better tracking of the patient's condition. Knowing where to allocate resources to prevent high-risk patients from requiring expensive, often unnecessary care means collecting data on patients and developing risk models that can identify high-risk patients earlier. Patients with multiple chronic conditions and medications or other signs that put them at high risk can then be targeted for additional care and interventions that help ensure compliance with drug regimens, lifestyle changes, remote monitoring, etc. And this means a lot of real-time data and patient-generated data are about to enter health systems beyond clinical or EHR data. Increasingly this will come from sensors in the home and a range of telehealth devices and population-based data sets that data scientists can use to understand individual risk files even better. Social determinants of health data also need to be rendered useful to clinicians and care managers so that the barriers to access in care and other social factors that often influence health outcomes even more than medical care can be integrated into treatment plans. Food deserts, for example, are a major factor leading to poor nutrition and exacerbated chronic disease conditions.

Data and the Quality of Care

For years a research team at Dartmouth has been collecting study of variations in practice patterns of physicians to understand widely varying patterns of care that emerge across the USA. The Dartmouth Atlas of Health Care is a treasure trove of insights into these practice patterns. The goal of the research is to understand what actually happens to patients and what can be done to improve the quality of care. There can be a twofold difference in Medicare spending from one region to another and little of the variation has to do with quality of care or outcomes. In fact, it is not uncommon to find the high-spending hospitals or physicians having worse outcomes associated with those practice patterns. And most of the difference is not a matter of high-utilization regions having sicker patients either. Furthermore, higher spending and more intensive utilization of services does not mean that people get healthier. Longer stays in hospitals, riskier procedures, and so forth can actually be bad for patients' health outcomes.[1] The research at

---

[1]http://www.dartmouthatlas.org/keyissues/issue.aspx?con=1338.

Dartmouth indicates that 20–30 % of all healthcare spending may be unnecessary. This is a pretty significant health policy problem with important public health consequences. It is widely viewed as up to 30 % of all care is unnecessary and data analytics will play a role in rationalizing care patterns in the coming years.

Additional research in the area of comparative effectiveness research illustrates just how hard it is to change medical practice even when there is an evidence base to support one procedure or medication over another. Comparative effectiveness research has been funded by the government to compare one treatment against another and determine the best treatment for a given illness. Despite the billions spent on the research over the years there is evidence that this has had little effect on changing clinicians' actual behaviors. A recent review of clinical practices published in the journal *Health Affairs* discovered a number of reasons why clinicians fail to act on what *these data* advise.[2] Some of the comparative effectiveness research was viewed by physicians as not responding sufficiently to the actual needs of clinicians. For example, one treatment may have better overall medical efficacy but the safety of the drug raised concerns for providers when the drug was compared to an alternative.[3] There were issues with some treatments requiring a different framing of the illness or treatment that was too marked a shift for both patients and doctors. But the most important factor boiled down to dollars. Studies that show that anything less that the most expensive or requiring anything less than the latest, greatest technology are often neglected and ignored. In a fee-for-service system lots of stakeholders gain from going after the latest, most expensive treatment. But the system, that means us, stands to gain when incentives are in alignment with the best procedure at the lowest cost. Marginal gains for substantial cost differentials—there have been few auditors looking over the shoulders of physicians to stop that kind of treatment. During the managed care period this type of thing provoked calls of rationing. Diuretic drugs that cost pennies per day and work better for high blood pressure are neglected out of a preference for the newest drugs that cost as much as 20 times more.[4] This type of practice has not serve the public well and the new regime that is coming down the pike might have some hope of changing this. New incentives for promoting value-based care, however, are beginning to change this type of practice. New platforms such as Castlight Health and HealthSparq help address part of this problem by creating more transparency for the consumer by providing cost and outcomes data by providers so that the "health consumer" can be better informed of the quality and costs of health services.

---

[2]http://healthaffairs.org/blog/2012/10/25/health-affairs-comparative-effectiveness-research-briefing-available-for-viewing/.

[3]http://well.blogs.nytimes.com/2012/11/08/why-studies-that-compare-treatments-lack-impact/?partner=rss&emc=rss.

[4]http://well.blogs.nytimes.com/2012/11/08/why-studies-that-compare-treatments-lack-impact/?partner=rss&emc=rss.

The challenges around improving the quality of care are only the tip of the data iceberg that is facing medicine in the coming years. In the introduction to the book we mentioned the challenge of the data deluge coming from research in the health and medical sciences. Physicians, health planners, and policy-makers must now wade through mountains of information to stay current with the standards of care, evidence base, and sheer volume of research. Frankly, it is no longer possible for human beings alone to handle the amount of new information. Whether you are a clinician or CFO of a hospital trying to integrate operational data with clinical data to inform your strategic plan, you have more data than you know what to do with. Patients can obviously collect their own data through tracking devices and bring in sheaths of research from their Google searches or health 2.0 community but how can all of these data be made actionable? Data analytics are coming to the forefront to help alleviate some of these problems. Before we go into some of the solutions that are out there we would like to take a brief detour so one can appreciate how the data deluge is only going to get worse with the growth of mobile sensors and the Internet of Things.

Sensors and the Internet of Things: The Health Internet of Things

The data deluge is about to get worse. Most of the wireless operators have made substantial investment in machine-to-machine (M2M) sensors, and health care is an important market for this service. Supply chains that supply hospitals and clinics with all of the drugs and operating supplies are increasingly monitored via sensors. Drugs need to be maintained at the proper temperatures and humidity to maintain a long shelf life. Patients have an increasing number of monitors that collect streaming, real-time data on their vital signs. Sensors can measure pollution levels (air, water, noise, weather) and are increasingly in the home as part of the medical home. The GSM Association estimates that by 2020 there will be 24 billion connected devices (2011 saw 9 billion) of which 12 billion will be mobile. These all collect data. Our automobiles over the next few years are likely to have sensors that can help you manage your asthma and have air sensors and other data collection technologies that will likely link to your mobile. Cities are collecting more data on traffic patterns, emissions, housing, walking indices, urban agricultural programs, and so on. Sensors, invisibly, are changing the physical world in some fundamental ways. The invisible patterns of our physical infrastructure are actually more visible than ever before. Smart cities, smart homes, wired patients, geo-location services that we use to check in, share data on what and where you are eating—these are the digital footprints that are coming together in the vast Internet of Things.

The Internet of Things refers to the use of sensors that are connected to the Internet and link the physical world with the virtual world. For many non-techies this may sound like something from the distant future but it is already well under way. Cisco has estimated that the number of connected things may reach 50 billion by 2020, much more than the 20 billion that GSMA predicts. In 2008 the number of things connected to the Internet surpassed the number of people for the first time.[5] Advances in nanotechnology are leading to sensors that we can embed in the body or on the body in the form of "tattoos" that can collect data and monitor physiological processes in the body, for example. These health-related sensors are part of what we call "the health Internet of Things" that is going to have a major impact on health care in the future. Already we have sensors connected to pill bottles that can detect if a patient has taken a pill at the correct time in alignment with the adherence regimen. Vitality has developed the Glowcaps technology to address the problem of the fact that over 50 % of prescriptions in the USA are either left unfilled or taken improperly resulting in a tremendous amount of waste. Slippers with sensors that can detect an elderly person's location in the house and whether they may have suffered a fall are going to be offered by AT&T shortly.

One of the more interesting emerging technologies in the health Internet of Things comes from a company originally called Asthmapolis, now renamed Propeller Health. According to the CDC approximately 14 people die per day due to asthma making it the 5th most expensive chronic disease to treat along with chronic obstructive pulmonary disorder at 6th most expensive. Asthma rates have also risen by over 30 % over the past two decades due to the rise of environmental pollution as we have become a more automobile-centric culture. Yet little is known about the contextual triggers about asthma because it is difficult to collect data at the precise moment when the asthmatic uses an inhaler. Propeller Health has developed a clever way to begin filling in the gaps in our public health knowledge and hopefully feed into community-based efforts to address the contextual triggers. They have developed a sensor that fits on the albuterol inhaler that is activated when an asthmatic is having an asthma attack. The sensor collects the geo-coordinate for the location. As more asthmatics begin using the device, they will be able to bring together environmental data and the asthma data to hopefully better understand environmental triggers. Other important sensor-driven projects that can help address important public health issues include the platform Xively (formerly Pachube then Cosm), sensor networks that were used in the wake of the 2011 Japanese Tsunami and Fukushima nuclear reactor crisis to create radiation maps. Sites such as Safecast.org, Radiation.crowdmap.com, or RDTN.org were used to crowdsource radiation sensor data to add greater transparency to the data released by the Japanese government. A similar use of sensors can be seen in China where the government is notoriously bad at providing accurate data on the air pollution levels associated with China's rapid industrialization process. The US Embassy has created their own iPhone/Android app that provides data from the sensors at the US Embassy that citizens can check for alternative readings. What is fascinating about a number of sensor projects is how citizens engage with the data. Andrew Barry has written about the experience in the UK when air pollution

---

[5]http://blogs.cisco.com/news/the-Internet-of-things-infographic/.

sensors were first used in the 1990s or British freeways and in London.[6] Public debate soon erupted over the data on specific pollutants and what levels of specific pollutants actually constituted a pollution threat.

The Internet of Things (IoT) is becoming a sector ripe for changing the way we deliver some health services. The government of China is acutely interested making use of sensors and has a healthcare budget of nearly $200 billion per annum,[7] and plans to spend over $600 billion by 2020 on the IoT industry alone. In 2010 the European Union endorsed the development of an IoT infrastructure. The endorsement also recognized the importance of frameworks for developing consumer trust in privacy and security for the IoT in healthcare systems.[8] Creating sufficient privacy and data governance policies will be increasingly important as the amount and types of data proliferate.

The need for data policies to support the growth of data collection and use was brought home by the World Economic Forum in 2011–12 as they issued a number of white papers and frameworks on health and personal data.[9] It is not uncommon to find data policies on the books that precede many of the technologies that are on the market and this creates a rather awkward situation. One illustrative example in the European Union happened when a Dutch company, Spark, developed sensors that could monitor the grazing habits of cattle. The sensor data were transmitted to the cloud but they came up against some policy hurdles when the data policies on the books for some countries stated that the servers for the data had to be in the country of data origin or this was a violation of data privacy protections. As cloud computing becomes the norm, we will need to have more informed discussions about privacy and security that can offer protections to consumers and companies but also enable innovation and data liquidity. These are often not easy to reconcile and many healthcare companies are still quite wary of the cloud but this is beginning to change. The first half of 2015 saw a number of very large hacking incidents such as the millions of records that were compromised at the largest insurer in the USA, Anthem. The World Economic Forum has highlighted the fact that the market value of personal data is increasing to the point where personal data are now a "new economic asset."[10] This fact is not lost on hackers and the value of health data on the dark Web appears to be increasing. By 2015 your stolen credit card data could be bought on the dark Web for one dollar per record but hacked health data went for $200–2000 depending on the type of health record.

WEF's efforts are focused on creating a global dialogue about personal data that will further an agenda constructed around a more user-centric framework for data policies where individuals will have more control over their data and how

---

[6]Andrew Barry, 2001. Political Machines. Governing a Technological Society. Athlone Press.

[7]http://www.chinadaily.com.cn/bizchina/2011-03/10/content_12151446.htm.

[8]http://www.readwriteweb.com/archives/parliament_of_things.php.

[9]The Health Data Charter offers a framework for rethinking health data policies in light of recent technological developments: http://www.weforum.org/issues/charter-health-data.

[10]World Economic Forum, 2011. Personal Data as a New Economic Asset. http://www.weforum.org/reports/personal-data-emergence-new-asset-class.

it is used as well as have means for compensation when their data are used for commercial gain. There may be a middle ground where data donation, data philanthropy, and data commons can be utilized for public goods research where the gains will be for public health and population health improvements or improving access to some medical services and goods. The Swiss startup company, healthbank mentioned earlier, is a model of how remunerative commons could be built to make more equitable data sharing arrangements.

In health care we are still a long way from data that are liquid and can flow across the system to the right people at the right time. Health information exchanges (HIEs) were developed to help address this problem and the regulatory environment for health technology in the USA has demanded greater interoperability from the EHR providers. Unfortunately, progress has been rather slow and the lack of progress is a growing political issue for some vendors. There is also a belief that until vendors get paid to address the problem that they will drag their feet. Value-based care demands the ability to exchange data readily but the transition to VBC will not happen overnight. One of the biggest improvements coming down the pike is the work done by health standards body HL7 to develop the Fast Healthcare Interoperability Resources (FHIR) and a collaboration of providers and health technology companies called Argonaut Project that will leverage APIs to dramatically improve data sharing across health systems.[11] Projects like this will need to accelerate to handle the amount of data that is coming from the more distributed sides of the healthcare sector as more patient-generated data and data from sensors explode.

If we think about this in the context of the IoT and a healthcare system more focused on prevention, we can reimagine new data services built on the IoT that are anticipatory and real-time in contrast to the retrospective approach of traditional medicine. No one has paid for prevention in the past, but we pay much more, a collective loss, for treating sickness downstream. Perverse incentives have prevented us from realizing the power of preventive approaches but that is beginning to change through value-based care. Esther Dyson offers an additional tool to provide incentives that will create greater investments in prevention. She offers a solution based on a "securitization" scheme for people's health. The paradox of prevention and market-led forces under-investing in prevention in the USA could be changed through this scheme. Her proposal involves assigning a monetary value to each person's health that would "securitize" intangible risks in a manner that gives an incentive to health plans to invest in prevention.[12] This would mean that a financial value would be assigned to a person's health. If the actual cost is less than predicted cost, the plan could make money through investment in prevention. Data analytics and health data value chains could form the backbone of this type of scheme when combined with the actuarial data that insurers already use to

---

[11]http://hl7.org/implement/standards/fhir/2015Jan/argonauts.html.

[12]David Bollier, 2010. The Promise and Peril of Big Data. Aspen Institute. http://www.aspeninstitute.org/publications/promise-peril-big-data.

run their business. Data analytics will not only serve the clinician and the healthcare system but can be brought into a relationship with open data and data commons to catalyze new ways of financing health care, or alternatively, wellness.

Data and the City

Much of the discussion on wireless health focuses on the medical home, the hospital, the clinic, and what transpires between a patient and a doctor. Perhaps more important is what goes on in our cities and how technology and data can help create a more prevention-focused healthcare system. To understand this better we may need to move beyond the typical healthcare system discussion to developments in urban planning, civic apps, and open data to see more clearly the potential of data. There is a great deal of innovation happening at the city level through open data programs that has actually inspired federal government initiatives aimed at making data more usable by citizens and entrepreneurs in the hope that pushing data out of silos or what former White House CTO Todd Parks calls "data vaults" could create the foundation for a new products and services. Park is well known for his data call to arms or "data liberacion!" as the new mantra for how government needs to open data catalogs and promote innovation.

To give you just one idea of how mobiles and passive data are helping to address problems at the city level, we can take a look at a simple, but very innovative app developed for the city of Boston. The interestingly named department of "New Urban Mechanics" created an app called Street Bump that residents can download on their phones.[13] As they drive through the city in their automobiles, the accelerometer can detect bumps in the street and the GPS maps where the bumps are located. As bumps are mapped on a server, the data are sent to the city's 311 service. The app was developed in partnership with Connected Bits (http://www.connectedbits.com/), a firm that develops apps for mobile reporters; InnoCentive, an open innovation platform; IDEO (design firm); and Fabio Carrera, an Italian university professor interested in data and cities. Why does this matter? For several decades we have known that the aesthetics and design of the built environment have social effects on how people perceive a neighborhood and civic engagement in maintaining a street. From Jane Jacob's work in the 1960s–70s in New York City to the Healthy Cities and Communities initiative created by the World Health Organization in the 1980s, there has been a steadily growing interest in the intersection of city planning and health. When roads begin to fail, this can have knock on effects and cause other parts of the urban community to begin to fracture as well. This is why some cities have aggressive anti-graffiti efforts that try to rid neighborhoods of some forms of graffiti that denote degradation of the city and promote street art that can build a sense of ownership. We can tell patients to exercise to control their diabetes but if they go home to communities with high

---

[13]http://www.newurbanmechanics.org/projects/streetscapes/bump/.

crime rates and no sidewalks the patient faces too many structural barriers to implement the preventive program. There are times when a new sidewalk is the best medicine.

An interesting illustration of how urban design, commerce and health can come together can be seen in Chicago in the mid-1990s. In mid-July 1995 a sudden heat wave hit Chicago. In the course of a week, power failed, residents had no air conditioning for several days leading to over 700 deaths. The death toll was greater than the toll from the 1871 Chicago Fire. A sociologist, Eric Klinenberg, conducted a "social autopsy" of the episode and uncovered some very interesting patterns in who died.[14] A combination of conditions in neighborhoods including aging demographics, poorly prepared public health authorities, and race leads to elderly African-Americans dying in the highest numbers. "Aging in place" had dire consequences when neighborhoods fraught with crime meant there was less street life and less cohesive social networks for elderly African-Americans when they needed access to these networks to gain access to cooling centers. Elderly Latinos died in much lower numbers due to more vibrant commercial street life in their neighborhoods that helped maintain these social networks. The social autopsy conducted by Klinenberg provides a compelling narrative about the "data" of city life and the social connections we need to maintain healthy neighborhoods. The technologies and data we have now can provide even more insights from the perspective of the macroscope of the city rather than the microscope of the clinic. Spatial intelligence will become an important asset for city planners, health planners and community organizations as maps, sensors, and data about urban life proliferate.

One such effort to map the data of city life and make sense of the diverse networks that can influence health outcomes is the work of the Senseable City Lab at MIT.[15] This is a laboratory created to study how digital technologies are changing the way we live and to understand the future of cities. Much akin to the Healthy Cities movement, they integrate urban planning, architecture, computer science, economics, to understand the effects of these technologies and then build applications that can provide solutions to urban problems. One of the research projects under way is a collaboration with GE called "Health Infoscape" that has analyzed anonymized electronic medical records (EMRs) of over 7.2 million patients. The goal is to map the relationships between space, geography, and health and explode our traditional, more isolated ways of thinking about disease and its boundaries.

---

[14]Eric Klinenberg, 2003. Heatwave: A Social Autopsy of Disaster in Chicago.

[15]http://senseable.mit.edu/.

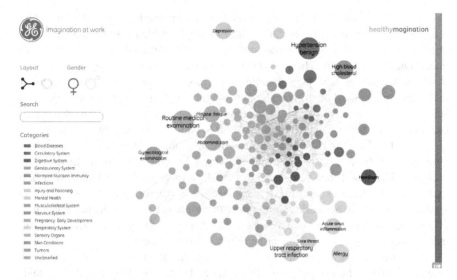

Health Infoscape: Senseable City Lab (MIT) and GE

Health Infoscape is an interactive map that lets one explore the connections between different diseases. Some of the connections may be familiar to readers but the aspect that many outside of health and medicine fail to appreciate is that the way we practice medicine has been largely based on studies that focus on one condition. The Health Infoscape visualization and much of the research on network effects and connections will help us to understand the complexity of health outcomes in a "real-world" sense rather than within the confines of a laboratory or controlled clinical trial. *We are living in an interesting historical moment where medicine and public health are moving from a retrospective form of medicine and public health to a more real-time, real-world view.* Data and technology are driving this change and it will have very profound implications for how we think about disease, communities and wellness in the future.

Social Network Analysis and Health Outcomes

Nicholas Christakis and James Fowler have been conducting studies that are a variant of this that looks at the impact of social networks on health outcomes.[16] Health outcomes may be less about individual choice than many of us think. The influence of social networks that we are all part of can be seen in things like

---

[16]Nicholas Christakis and James Fowler, 2011. Connected: The Surprising Power of our Social Networks and How they Shape Our Lives. Back Bay Books.

obesity rates, diabetes, and even death rates. These researchers took at a large data set used by health researchers called the Framingham Heart Study that followed individuals from 1971 to 2003 and analyzed social relationships and the connections to health outcomes. The researchers looked at the body mass index of participants in the study and then examined the social networks of each member including spouses, siblings, friends, and neighbors. What their research demonstrated was that a person's risk of becoming obese increased by 57 % if a friend became obese in a given time interval. If a sibling became obese one's risk increased by 40 and 37 % if a spouse became obese. Depression has similar dynamics. If friends in your social networks become depressed, there is an increased likelihood that you may become depressed as well.[17] Depression and many chronic diseases may have very important network effects and actually spread through our networks. Sometimes these effects are due to the contagion effect—that is, they spread like a disease. In other cases the convergence to a norm may be more an effect of socialization of a behavior or norm.

There are other ways of understanding network effects and health as well. A research group at the University of Rochester called the "Healthy Insights in Real-Time" uses big data analytics and artificial intelligence or machine learning tools to understand social networks and health issues through analytics of social media. This research group utilizes machine learning and natural language processing (NLP) to extract insights from Twitter in real-time. This has proven useful in tracking outbreaks of infectious diseases as people discuss their symptoms on Twitter. The data on Twitter are useful for health researchers because it is open data that can be mined using computing tools and tweets contain time and date stamps. By mining Twitter for tweets containing content on flu symptoms, asthma or allergies or foodborne illnesses they can create heat maps that display densities of tweets containing a particular symptom. From these heat maps they can dive even deeper for a more granular analysis of individual tweets and the person's connections to other individuals containing similar symptoms. From this type of social network analysis of Twitter and health they can generate real-time analytics of how different social networks interact. In 2010 they noticed symptoms of a foodborne illness outbreak in New York City. Typically it takes the media weeks and even months to identify the source of a salmonella outbreak. Using their artificial intelligence tools and Twitter they were able to identify the source of the outbreak 10–12 days sooner than the Centers for Disease Control and Prevention who utilize more traditional disease surveillance tools based on clinical records. Tools such as this and platforms like Google's Flu Trends (http://www.google.org/flu-trends/), FluNearYou (https://flunearyou.org/), and SickWeather (http://www.sick-weather.com/) offer a new paradigm for conducting disease surveillance that could allow public health officials to intervene much sooner and contain outbreaks. In early 2016 SickWeather accurately predicted the week that seasonal influenza would peek nearly 3 months before the event. The research team at the University of Rochester has been able to generate predictive models that are predictive of

---

[17]http://jhfowler.ucsd.edu/social_network_determinants_of_depression.pdf.

when people in specific areas are likely to get sick with an accuracy rate of 90 %.[18]

We can also turn to developing countries for some insights into how real-time mapping and reporting of health issues is taking advantage of open data and crowdsourcing. In 2008 when Kenya was on the verge of a major national election, ethnic violence broke out around the country. The government, in an effort to control the situation, demanded a media ban on reporting about the violence. A number of political bloggers felt that this would not help the situation and began using their blogs to report on incidents of violence. Soon technologists such as Erik Hersman, a Kenyan raised in both Sudan and Kenya, came to the assistance of the bloggers and built an open-source platform that allowed people to send SMS messages or tweets indicating an outbreak of violence or a counterviolence episode. These could be mapped on the platform and create a visualization of the situation on the ground. The platform was named "Ushahidi," a Swahili word for "testimony" or "to testify." Since 2008 the Ushahidi platform has been used all over the world to map human rights abuses, harassment of women in Cairo and even as a civic app in Washington, DC during the 2009 blizzard where it allowed people to map streets that had not been plowed so that community members could work together to clear the streets. The experience of Ushahidi helped highlight the beneficial aspects of transparency and opening up data and communities of activists began to advocate for an expansion of efforts. This eventually led to one of the most secretive and closed international development organizations, the World Bank, to become one of the leading advocates for governments to open up data and let people build applications and services that can benefit the public and overall development efforts.

We can see further evidence of the impact of Ushahidi and mobiles in the area of disaster recovery in the wake of the 2010 earthquake in Haiti. By then we had seen Twitter used during wildfires in California and for hurricane preparedness. Earthquake recovery efforts require a different level of assistance than election monitoring or human rights reporting. What is needed is a way to coordinate complex relief operations. In order to pull this off a team of "crisis mappers" based in Boston worked with others in the emerging Ushahidi network of techies focused on humanitarian issues. This involved organizations like the Palo Alto-based nonprofit InSTEDD that was seasoned in humanitarian relief as well as mHealth tools for data collection and coordination of logistics in South East Asian health systems and emergencies. As Andrew Zolli points out, this was a loose network of organizations and individuals collaborating rather than the usual UN humanitarian relief operation that tends to be more hierarchical, and for many, not as effective as they could be within the command-and-control hierarchies that dominate UN efforts.[19]

Other members of the network worked with the Haitian government and wireless carriers to get a shortcode that Haitians with mobiles could use to report

---

[18]ibid.

[19]Andrew Zolli and Ann Marie Healy, 2012. Resilience. Why Things Bounce Back. Free Press, pp. 177–183. Note: one author, Jody Ranck, worked with InSTEDD from 2010 to 2011.

information or call in emergencies. This would be like a 311 code used by cities in the USA. Digicel, the largest telco in Haiti, provided a 4636 number for Haitians to use. This was one of the initial steps needed to coordinate action. The other challenge was the lack of accurate maps and street addresses in Port-au-Prince, the capital. Volunteers were assembling at Tufts University and around the world to map data as it came in and with groups of expat Haitians who could translate texts messages from Kreyol (Creole) while InSTEDD worked to put into place the backend technological infrastructure that could pull all of the streams of data together and route information out to disaster recovery personnel. This ad hoc system of technology and volunteers processed more than 10,000 SM messages, sometimes reaching 5000 messages processed in one hour.[20] Countless lives were saved.

We provide the example of Ushahidi to shed light on how open platforms, social networks and emerging technologies can make a major difference even in places where the basic technological infrastructure is weak. Furthermore, we believe that the technologies that are being deployed in health are networking technologies that have deep implications for how we will organize our health systems. However, for the most part, policy-makers and planners are still thinking in analog terms. We have network technologies and tools like social network analysis that can offer new ways of thinking about the spread of diseases but also offer insights on how we might be able to reconfigure hospitals, cities, networks of care and even how we fund health care. We have network technologies but are still working with analog institutions.

The success of Ushahidi and open data projects has inspired the notion of "government or city as platform" as coined by technology publisher Tim O'Reilly.[21] This is a way of rethinking the role of government in providing new products and services that harnesses the power of web 2.0 platforms and the ability to engage with the public, entrepreneurs and users of government services in new ways. The role of the citizen is more active and the platforms are meant to provide the tools that people can use to build new tools that promote greater civic engagement, improve city life or health outcomes, for example. It also is a marked shift, in many ways, from the past in that transparency is embraced and data, rather than being in the hands of government researchers or those with PhDs, are put into a format that is easier to use, machine-readable (app-friendly). Cloud computing is also part of the equation and becomes a tool to make the various parts of government that typically just fight over turf find ways to share data and resources. The federal government created Data.gov as a site for anyone to gain access to data that the government has collected. Parallel to Data.gov is Challenge.gov where you can find the latest innovation challenges that frequently involve taking data sets and then building an app or service based on these data. The cloud is creating the conditions for interesting uses of computing that lean toward

---

[20]Ibid, p. 185.

[21]http://www.slideshare.net/timoreilly/government-as-platform.

Infrastructure-as-a-Service that offers more consumer-friendly ways of offering computing to large numbers of people or organizations when they need it.

At the city level we can find both private and public types of platforms that are emerging to address public goods such as health. From platforms like See Click Fix (http://www.seeclickfix.com/) to Neighbor.ly (http://neighbor.ly/) (a platform that functions like Kickstarter (http://www.kickstarter.com/) but for projects at the city scale) the notion of city as a platform or government 2.0 is beginning to take hold and could become a driving force for innovation at the nexus of data, health and mobiles in the coming years. Other non-governmental organizations (NGOs) are focusing on building the data and technological literacies required for fruitful engagement with these platforms. Organizations like the School of Data (http://schoolofdata.org/) help teach people how to find and use data and build useful apps. Hackathons, many of them geared toward developing apps that have a public health focus are coming out of many of these efforts.

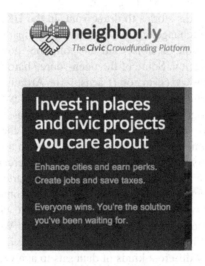

Over the years we have presented trends in the area of open data, mHealth and open innovation, many health professionals in the audience have spoken up immediately to raise their concerns about the quality of data, research outputs and the scientific method when they hear about these efforts. Often what they fail to realize is that the early efforts in these areas have demonstrated that the more people use data, the better the data become. More eyeballs means more cross-checking and even scrutiny of the categories used for data collection. On occasion the categories used by government or researchers are dated and have little sociological relevance to the social worlds that people inhabit. Furthermore, medical scientists and public health researchers often overestimate the power of their own scientific method. We need only go back to stories of the search for the cause of gastric ulcers. When researchers Barry Marshall and J. Robert Warren first postulated that ulcers had an infectious agent, *helicobacter pylori*, as the cause of ulcers, they were treated as quacks by the medical research profession. Lo and behold, in 1995 they were awarded the Nobel Prize in Medicine.[22] Any public health professional knows that one of the biggest public health challenges is to get the public to pay attention to new public health research. One of the reasons, one could argue, is that the public has become accustomed to epidemiologists releasing the results of one study indicating a causal relationship that x produces y health outcome and then a year later another study repudiating this. On average, health policy experts feel that it takes approximately eight years from the time an initial study is done until one can make policy on the basis of that study given the way that science currently works. This costs a lot of lives and money in some cases. One can make a strong argument that utilizing crowdsourcing tools, mobile infrastructures, the cloud and more engaged citizen scientists who have demonstrated the ability through projects such as Foldit (http://www.fold.it/) and CellSlider (http://www.cellslider.net/) (a UK-based platform that crowdsources the identification of tumor cells in suspected cancer cell biopsies) that alternative models of production of scientific knowledge could be what we need.

There are many success stories to draw from. In the UK, Mapping for Change (http://www.mappingforchange.org.uk/) has used participatory mapping to engage citizens in data collection on noise and air pollution, government spending on infrastructure and education. Some of the open-source hardware projects based on Pachube/Cosm (http://www.cosm.com/) sensors or Arduino components that we have spoken about earlier have achieved levels of complexity that are quite fascinating.[23] One Kickstarter Project even includes a DIY mass spectrometer.[24] Public Lab, a citizen science platform, wanted to create a cheap spectrometer that attaches to a smart phone that the average person can use for monitoring pollution levels and contaminants in their own backyards. Commercial mass spectrometers cost hundreds and even thousands of dollars. The Kickstarter campaign is focused on developing a $35 device that is as accurate as most commercial devices. They also focus on the software and the development of what will be the Open Street Map of spectral data from the devices called the Spectral Workbench (http://spectralworkbench.org/). When you have enough users of the device and the software we can then have many different kinds of data sets to analyze in typical "big data" fashion. There are other examples of how platforms for data collection and massive data collection by laypersons may make an impact in medical research. A recently launched effort in the area of cardiology at the University of Southern California will be interesting to watch in the coming years. Leslie Saxon, from the Center for Body Computing (http://uscbodycomputing.org/), specializes in wearable computing devices for cardiology research. She has been working with the entertainment industry to come up with ways that data collection about the body can be gamified and devices such as Alivecor's cardiac monitoring system could be popularized to collect real-time data on millions, perhaps billions of individuals

---

[22]http://www.nobelprize.org/nobel_prizes/medicine/laureates/2005/press.html.

[23]www.internetartizans.co.uk/bigdatacapability.

[24]http://www.pbs.org/idealab/2012/09/public-lab-uses-kickstarter-to-bring-diy-spectrometry-to-the-masses254.html.

and help us understand heart disease in ways that we have been unable to study it in the past. These are just some of the ways that the conditions for big data takeoff in the health and medical sciences are getting ready for takeoff.

Data Analytics and Health care

The business world is rife with chatter and hype about big data these days. As with most technology trends, big data certainly has to contend with a lot of hyperbole about the latest quest for the holy grail. But the importance of data analytics in health care is very real and is only going to grow as we gradually shift to a more value-based healthcare economy. Data analytics will play a part in addressing inefficiencies and fraud, improving clinical practice, and making sense of all the data collected on sensors and devices. Increasingly the think tanks and health policy crowd is recognizing that we need to make the healthcare system more data-driven and performance-oriented. In April 2012 the Kauffman Task Force on Cost-Effective Health Care Innovation released their findings on a research endeavor that sought to answer: How can we get a lot more bang for the buck in health care?[25] The Task Force framed this in terms of how to "unlock" or "jailbreak" existing resources such as organizational skills, knowledge and resources of patients. The Key to jailbreaking health care or transforming the healthcare system will be to utilize information, improve collaboration and empower patients. Data will be an important factor in each one of the steps.

What do we mean by big data? We typically find big data defined in terms of the "3 Vs":[26]

- **Volume**: The volume of data has moved beyond a single server or terabytes to petabytes, zettabytes, and beyond.
- **Variety**: Traditional research focused primarily on structured data and the cost in terms of time and money for analyzing unstructured data was high. Some big data tools have lowered the cost of analyzing unstructured data. The growth of use of social media in health care has resulted in a new type of unstructured data for healthcare analytics.
- **Velocity**: Big data platforms have the capacity to analyze streaming or real-time data from a large number of devices. The health Internet of Things and M2M are contributing to more streaming data from medical devices throughout hospitals. Passive monitoring from mobiles and sensors, for example, are demanding the capacity for real-time processing of data.

The fourth V that has been added more recently is **Veracity**. Provenance of data and data quality are always going to be of central importance in health care. Provenance and security are also important areas where innovations such

---

[25]http://www.kauffman.org/uploadedfiles/valuing_health_care.pdf.

[26]See Jody Ranck (2012). Big Data and Healthcare. GigaOm Research.

as Blockchain may make inroads in health care. Blockchain is a cryptographic, distributed ledger system that the alternative currency Bitcoin is built upon. It is useful as a way to track provenance of data while also maintaining high levels of security. Of growing value in the financial sector, I expect that we will see innovations for creating new types of research commons that incentivize patients to share data, enabling researchers to ascertain the provenance of the data, while also giving the patient the ability to control who accesses their data through the use of multi-signature keys that are part of the Blockchain infrastructure. Blockchain can also help address the challenge of maintaining anonymity through the cryptographic layer it would provide in medical research commons and MIT has a research group that recently developed Enigma, a Blockchain-based anonymization layer. While we are still in the early days, it will be interesting to monitor emerging Blockchain and healthcare applications in the coming years.

In 2011 the power of big data was brought home to a popular audience when IBM's Watson went face-to-face with Brad Rutter, the all-time leading winner on the popular game show Jeopardy! who had won over $3.4 million. For the competition Watson had access to 200 million pages of structured and unstructured text that amounted to four terabytes of storage.[27] The computing power of IBM's Watson is such that it can tear through this amount of data in seconds, even milliseconds, to generate an answer to a question. The big question for Watson Health is going to be how to integrate the right analytics into healthcare organizations in a manner that will change organizational and clinician behavior to optimize health outcomes and save money.

Data analytics companies came about due to the needs of some of the biggest companies driving the growth of the Internet requiring substantial computing power capable of data mining at Web scale. Google and Yahoo created open-source tools out of Apache code that could parse data on many serial servers in a manner that would not fail, or break down easily when running large batches of data. The two most popular tools are Hadoop and Map Reduce. Google and Yahoo need to be able to cope with the current load of about 2.5 quintillion bytes of data produced daily. It is not only the volume of these data that is the challenge but the type of data can create difficulties for data scientists wanting to make sense of the sheer volume. Unstructured data that is not collected via structured or coded surveys has always been an expensive and time-consuming data challenge. NLP and machine learning are part of the big data set of tools that has been one of the disruptive innovations in computing that generates much of the excitement about big data. The vast amounts of data generated on Twitter and Facebook would be a huge challenge for marketers to do anything with if we did not have big data to help us analyze unstructured data.

Health care is in a similar boat in respect of the data deluge and unstructured data. We are in the early days of adopting EMRs and reached about half of all physician practices utilizing EHRs in 2012. In mid-2015 nearly 70 % of medical

---

[27]http://en.wikipedia.org/wiki/Watson_(computer).

practices had adopted EHRs. But still we have approximately 80 % of health data in unstructured formats that are difficult to analyze without the use of NLP tools. This is not the medical profession's fault but a matter of how medicine has been practiced traditionally. Furthermore, most data are stuck within legacy health IT systems in hospitals that do not interoperate easily and this is even becoming a political issue. That means when you get your laboratory tests that those data may not go directly to the system where your medical records exist. The clinical data may not readily work with the financial data system that the hospital uses. Now, imagine you go from your primary care physician to a specialist. Remember the hassle of getting your records to the specialist or to the hospital and the need to recount your story over and over again. Why can't the original set of data just be integrated? Well, we are dealing with an antiquated and siloed health system and health data standards that are still falling short. Despite regulatory requirements for improved interoperability, progress is extremely slow due to the business models of legacy technology players. These technologies are typically pre-Internet technologies that are ill-equipped for Web-based approaches to computing. The new HL7 standard, FHIR, is expected to help health care catch up to other parts of the economy, but we will likely not see anything resembling Amazon or Google for health care for at least another 5–10 years.

We would also like to make one thing clear—data are going to drive a lot of the transformation in the digital health era, but it is not the only game in town. The Quantified Self is a fascinating and important trend that has the potential to enhance our understanding of the body. But if we reduce the body to the data that can quantify vitals and so on we can miss other, equally important dimensions of the body and health. We have to be careful not to get caught up in the hubris of exciting technological trends. Likewise, big data can help us to create a much more efficient system but we need organizational innovations to match the power of networking technologies. Policy innovations that can keep up with our knowledge of health and the technologies we use to manage our health will need to happen as well. The current frameworks for assessing technologies and reimbursing healthcare professionals who use them are dated. When we hear venture capitalists such as Vinod Khosla make claims that algorithms are going to render 80 % of physicians obsolete, we need to take this with a grain of salt. Perhaps a better way of stating this would be that 80 % of the unproductive time that doctors and nurses spend doing paperwork or researching a disease so that they can come up with a better diagnosis—these tasks may be replaced by technologies and algorithms. Business models built on the old fee-for-service model that has become incredibly inefficient; these may be facing disruptive models in the coming years. Medicine and public health still require substantial human-to-human interaction. The technologies we are talking about here are tools for better patient safety, system efficiencies, clinical decision support, operational efficiencies, fraud detection, early outbreak detection, and so on. This is where we expect to see some major gains in the coming years and we will offer some windows into the power of big data below.

IBM through their big data suite of tools such as Watson, Netezza, and collaborations with academic medical centers is one of the largest players in the field. But the shift to value-based care has made data analytics offering a robust sector in the overall health economy. Population health management demands real-time data analytics and many health IT vendors are competing to offer tools for providers to monitor population health outcomes. But it is still the early days and marketing rhetoric often outpaces the ability to deliver results. There is a great deal of research that IBM is doing in the realm of cancer biology and therapeutics that could are bringing personalized medicine closer to reality. IBM collaborates with the Sloan Kettering Center on one project that illustrates the nature of research in this area.[28] The idea is to take the data analytics potential of IBM's Watson to the molecular and genomic databases that the clinical researchers at Sloan Kettering have created with researchers worldwide and be able to scan the standards of care and published data alongside patient health records to develop tools that can customize cancer therapies to individual biologies. Often when a patient undergoes chemotherapy for cancer there is a period of trial and error with various medications until the right drug cocktail can be optimized for a particular patient's individual characteristics. Personalized medicine will enable the targeting of therapies to happen faster. The National Cancer Institute has already developed a tool that taps into the vast amount of data on cancer to help patients and clinicians decide which course of therapy is best for a patient given their general health status and other factors. The tool, MyCancerGenome.org is built on the existing literature on cancer and allows patients and providers to model different treatments and life expectancies and probabilities of success. It is a worldwide collaborative effort that involves 40 researchers and 13 medical research institutions.

Getting back to IBM, they are also involved with research on multiple sclerosis through a collaboration with the State University of New York at Buffalo.[29] Multiple sclerosis (MS) is a rather idiosyncratic disease where individual patients can have very different sets of symptoms that make it a bit tricky for physicians to develop an effective therapy. Furthermore, scientists have noticed a gradient in the prevalence of MS that follows a North–South continuum with higher rates of MS in the colder, more northern climates and lower prevalence rates in warmer climates. This observation has raised a question for researchers on whether there are environmental drivers of MS. Could sunlight, diet, vitamin D, or some combination of the above be connected to the gradient? IBM is using their Netezza platform with SUNY-Buffalo researchers to study up to 2000 genomic and environmental factors that may lie at the heart of this scientific puzzle. Genome–environment interactions are extremely complex, but understanding these interactions could enable physicians to customize treatment for MS sufferers before damage is done to the nervous system.

---

[28]http://www.mskcc.org/blog/mskcc-and-ibm-will-collaborate-powerful-new-medical-technology.

[29]http://www.eweek.com/c/a/Health-Care-IT/IBM-Revolution-Analytics-Speed-Up-MS-Research-at-SUNY-Buffalo-330317/.

Another important area that is going to become a big ticket issue for hospitals in the coming years is nosocomial infections. Hospital-acquired infections, particularly pneumonia, and *Staphylococcus aureus* infections (MRSA especially) are quite dangerous infections. In adults who become infected with any form of pneumonia pathogen in the hospital face the likelihood that 50 % of the time the antibiotic initially used will not be effective. Getting the wrong antibiotic in the first few days after diagnosis increases the likelihood of mortality by close to 50 %. This also increases the length of stay in a hospital substantially costing upwards of $20,000 each time a case is misdiagnosed, much less the risk of dying. Therefore many lives can be saved, suffering and substantial costs avoided by detecting the right pathogen as soon as possible. One can imagine that this problem is magnified in newborn infants whose immune systems are not fully developed. IBM has been working with clinical researchers on an interesting project in exactly this area that can help save the lives of infants. Earlier we mentioned remote monitoring devices and M2M technologies that are being deployed in the home and hospital to monitor patients. In the past, hospitals have kept the data from remote monitoring technologies in neonatal wards for up to three days and then the data were destroyed. Nurses and physicians in neonatal wards have been trained to focus on the alerts that go off when the monitoring tools detect an outlier data point. Here is where big data and data analytics can make a difference. Cloud storage and analytics tools such as IBMs enable researchers to collect real-time, streaming data for longer periods of time beyond the traditional three-day window. They can then analyze these data in relationship to health outcomes of neonates. Researchers working with IBM have done precisely this and made discoveries around subtle changes in heart rates of neonates that are an indication of the early onset of bacterial infections. The changes were too subtle for clinicians to observe in the course of their very hectic workflows in the neonatal wards. Something that had been invisible is now visible thanks to some technology and data analytics.

The reach of big data is not just in the clinical and research arenas. We can look at the work that LexisNexis Risk Solutions is doing in the healthcare arena to see how big data and population-based data can improve system efficiencies and meet the challenge of fraud. Inefficiencies and fraud, you might recall, cost the US healthcare system approximately $750 billion annually. LexisNexis Risk Solutions has developed the capacity to use large public records sets and data models. Some of their models have focused on social networks of Medicare fraud, for example, identifying clusters of Medicare recipients and assets (e.g., expensive cars) that are early warning signals. More interesting from a health outcomes perspective is their ability to create indices on neighborhoods for walkability, social cohesiveness, and strength of face-to-face networks. Data models on neighborhood characteristics can be invaluable for disease management and elder care interventions. These models enable planners to identify neighborhoods where social supports are weak and supplemental interventions may be needed to ensure compliance with behavioral changes and medication adherence programs, for example. When you look at the confluence of participatory mapping, passive sensing, and big data, we can begin to see how new research questions may arise out of big data efforts in the coming years. What if diabetes and other chronic diseases have more "social" dimensions than we had previously thought due to the prevalence of narrow bio-medically oriented research design that has dominated the medical sciences for decades? Big data represents a new social science opportunity to bridge the gap between the biological sciences, city planning and big data in ways that could enrich the science of prevention.

The Healthy Communities Initiative is a public health effort that uses data from government sources to help NGOs and communities create data dashboards on their local level health indicators. The indicators include data on poverty, housing, county health rankings, exercise, food safety, immunization rates, and so on. In addition, they have databases about best practices from community-based organizations that have created programs and services around these data. Here we see how data can become a rallying point for local organizations and stakeholders to build new collaborations to address the problems that the data speak to. Just as the new ACOs will need to use data as the glue to build a network of care to maintain the continuity of care, community-based organizations will increasingly be able to use population-based data for networked approaches that can address complex problems rather than the single solution approach that so often dominates local public health efforts. Networks of population-based care may also help build more resilient systems in the future. Data analytics will play a big role here.

There are some early examples of big data and grassroots responses to public health problems as well. Datakind works with DC Action for Children to assess well-being of children in the District of Columbia and uses data to help build the common language across policy-makers, citizens and child advocates.[30] One of the more successful community-based approaches to data analytics has been the work pioneered by Dr. Jeffrey Brenner who founded the Camden Coalition of Healthcare Providers. After analyzing ER admissions, hospital billing data, and local crime reports he identified individuals who were the "super-utilizers" of the ER, the locations of the super-utilizers, and the gaps in social services. For example, thirteen percent of patients accounted for eighty percent of hospital costs and twenty percent of patients accounted for ninety percent of the healthcare expenditures.[31] The database evolved into a HIE used by the local hospitals. These data were then used to foster the formation of patient management program that focuses on the following:

- Creation of a database to identify the super-utilizers
- Development of care management teams that use a nurse, social worker, community health worker and a health coach (AmeriCorps volunteer) who plan for the discharge and visit the home of the patient while coordinating with doctors and nurses for nine months after the discharge

---

[30]http://www.fastcoexist.com/1680931/the-potential-of-data-and-human-capital-to-change-the-world?partner=rss.

[31]http://www.rwjf.org/en/library/articles-and-news/2014/02/improving-management-of-health-care-superutilizers.html.

- Creation of a similar approach to care transition team to lower the risk of readmissions

The initial evaluation of the program not only demonstrated improvements in care but savings to Medicaid from a reduction in spending from $1.2 million to $500,000 in the first year. The program and the methodology of "hotspotting" have been focusing on replication and scaling the impact to other communities. Some of the key features of the methodology from a data analytics perspective include the following[32]:

- Use of real-time data and reports from the HIE that provide daily reports to care management teams
- A focus on filling in the gaps on social, contextual data on crime, housing, and bringing community organizations together to share data

In the current environment using data analytics to bridge the gap across care coordinators, the clinic and the community will be vital to managing chronic conditions in an aging population.

Pharmaceutical companies are beginning to utilize analytics and mobile applications to move beyond merely producing pills. In the coming years big data will be used to create better designed clinical trials that can target the right patients for better results in trials and to avoid costly failure late in the clinical trials process that adds substantially to the overall price of drugs. The era of slightly modifying the molecular structure of a compound without demonstrating a contribution to better outcomes is over. Pharmaceutical companies will need to come to the table with new types of data that can demonstrate outcomes and what the overall cost of managing a disease will be rather than only offering a drug with a price tag. This is part of the rationalization of health care that will be a painful transition for many players when they are now held accountable for costs and quality of care.

Privacy and Ethics in the Era of Data Analytics

We will also encounter many obstacles along the way. Researchers have used big data tools to large anonymized health data sets and combined these with cell phone records and other data to de-anonymize individuals. This poses a major privacy threat and our policy frameworks will need to come to terms with these challenges. Having sensors in the home means we will have the ability to track things that people would prefer not be tracked. We live in a pluralistic society where cultural norms differ across society and who gets to "see" what and where will come up against the power of the technology. Nano-sensors in the body that monitor our drug compliance or lifestyle choices will be viewed as a threat to civil liberties if it

---

[32]http://www.chcs.org/hotspotting-driver-behind-camden-coalitions-innovations/.

means one can end up paying more for insurance. Risky behaviors right now mean that we all end up paying for these behaviors. In an era where individual choice often dominates we can expect to find clashes in these norms and who determines what works for whom. In the 1990s many were alarmed at the privacy risks with genetics but we now have genetics plus sensors and analytics.

One way to address some of these concerns is for the public to understand the benefits. If technologists and health policy-makers just assume everyone gets why we are excited by health IT, they may be in for a rude awakening. One of the goals of writing this book is to help address technological literacies when it comes to health and to provoke intelligent debate about the choices we have to make in the coming years. More participatory policy approaches and using the technologies for public benefit, like many of the organizations discussed here are attempting to realize, may open up other avenues for engaging the public in spirited and informed discussions about technologies and data. As one prominent technology blogger recently stated it, big data may be the civil rights issue of our age, we just do not know it yet.[33] With the growing number of privacy and security breaches affecting health data, sometimes numbering in the tens of millions of patient records, trust will become a primary currency in digital health going forward. This will require industry-wide cooperation to build the standards and policies that can support the sharing of data, patient engagement, and security. Managing the tension between privacy and sharing will be critical to unlocking the value of health data for patients. It would be best to create forums where technologists, healthcare professionals, and the public could engage in a proactive and constructive manner about new policy frameworks that can keep pace with the rate of technology change; therefore at healthbank we are developing a Health Data Lab to create an international forum for precisely these types of activities so that the collective value of our health data can be leveraged for the public good.

A final way to approach data and build trust is through the nascent movement to build Data Collaboratives. A number of telecommunications companies in Europe and Africa, for example, have made anonymized cell phone data available for data scientists to analyze trends. Some of the studies are looking at how we can track the spread of diseases from combining cell phone data with epidemiological surveillance data to build models for the movements of people and diseases. UN Global Pulse collects data from NGO evaluations and data collection efforts with data from weather and agricultural extension programs to develop early warning systems for food security crises. Similar efforts can be adapted to the US context for understanding urban food deserts, for example. One can take the example of DMC International as an interesting model for data sharing that we could appropriate in health care.[34] DMCii is a private firm that handles large databases of satellite imagery and makes these readily available to countries or regions during severe weather events and crises. Twitter offers Data Grants that enable real-time

---

[33] http://solveforinteresting.com/big-data-is-our-generations-civil-rights-issue-and-we-dont-know-it/ and http://solveforinteresting.com/followup-on-big-data-and-civil-rights/.

[34] https://hbr.org/2014/07/sharing-data-is-a-form-of-corporate-philanthropy/.

access to their data to researchers who could use the data to monitor disease outbreaks or foodborne illnesses, for example. Intel shares satellite data with university researchers to better understand snowfall in the Sierra Nevada mountains that provide some of the primary water resources for coastal California. We should not be surprised to find that in the near future weather, air quality, pollen counts, and numerous other environmental data sets become part of health data analytics offerings and are rendered into actionable intelligence for patients and providers as they collaborate to manage diseases. This will transform medicine as we now know it.

There are many barriers for data sharing for the public good, however. Many companies and governmental departments view their data as strategic assets that are key to their competitive advantage or turf. Getting organizations to move from short-term thinking to longer term gains is often a serious challenge but it is possible to create tools used in building new commons to get organizations to shift perspectives. Data standards and different data protection measures can also impede sharing of data or the ability to integrate data. Who benefits is another question and can we rethink policies to reward data sharing. In health systems right now when it comes to the large EHR providers who are accused of "data blocking" we need to ask who gets paid or rewarded for data sharing when we think of regulatory and reimbursement policies. This will be incredibly important in the coming years. Those who advocate for data collaborations will need to become astute at communicating the wider social benefits, branding opportunities, and the return on investment (ROI) for the major players involved or targeted to participate. Realistic views of the dangers to privacy weighed against the opportunities for medical or health benefit also need to be considered along with ways to remedy those that could be harmed by privacy breaches.

One final note is that to build a collaborative data sharing ecosystem for health we need to become better stewards of the commons. Insurers, for example, could share data to build much more effective healthcare delivery systems but their competitive advantage is built around their actuarial science they run on top of their data. Finding a trusted third party that could act as a neutral player and govern the rules of the road for data sharing and avoid unfair advantages to one player over another is a necessary piece of the puzzle that is currently missing. With greater consolidation in the health payer market in the USA it is questionable whether data sharing is a reality depending on how competitive market forces line up in the coming years but there is a great deal of good that could be done from cooperation across payer, provider, pharma, and government and community-based organization lines if trust could be developed and a mission to unlock data for better health outcomes could be framed in a way and governed so that all parties gain, especially the public. We are beginning to see more movement on this front in pharma with some companies sharing data from clinical trials. There is much good that could be done from sharing data to fill in our scientific and public health knowledge gaps and then players compete for the best solution to address the problem. This will require a great deal of policy innovation to create the foundations for cooperation.

Chapter 7
Delivery of Digital Health Care Solutions—A Complex Challenge

Sven Schuchardt

In order for digital health offerings to be worthy of the investment, they must have an evidence base that demonstrates their contribution to improving health outcomes, their cost-effectiveness and have the ability to demonstrate improvements in quality of care. For telecommunications and digital service providers, this translates into requirements for scalability and performance and quality management. All these performance indicators are challenged by cost, quality, and availability of the delivered service.

This chapter focuses on the actual delivery of the digital health service from a telecommunications provider's perspective. In this world, the patient's information and his medical records are captured by the notion of a digital payload. It is paramount that these data are of highest quality and integrity and access to the data and service must be governed by strict policies to ensure that only those with legitimate medical reasons or those having the consent of the patient can access the data. On first glance, it would appear as though a digital health service is a very specific and custom-tailored service since it is designed to support the treatment path of a patient's specific condition.

A typical example is the remote monitoring of heart rate and blood pressure of cardiovascular patients. The patient uses specific devices at home that automatically transfer the data to a central telemedical center. In the medical center, the data are reviewed on a regular basis by the medical personnel in charge of the patient. The data collection and monitoring service may be combined with on call service of mobile nurses, regular checkups via telephone, reminders for medication, potentially linkage into other rehabilitation activities, and even data analysis services.

S. Schuchardt (✉)
Detecon International GmbH, Munich, Germany
e-mail: sven.schuchardt@detecon.com

© Springer International Publishing Switzerland 2016
J. Ranck (ed.), *Disruptive Cooperation in Digital Health*,
DOI 10.1007/978-3-319-40980-1_7

The above description of the service looks quite comprehensive. But we need to look deeper to guarantee the integrity of the service. The description above describes only the service operations and focuses very much on the care of one single patient. This may be perfectly suited from a medical point of view since it covers all data collection and intervention points to sufficiently control and improve the patient's health status. But we are living in an era of population health management and we need to build systems with the capacity to monitor much larger populations of patients where each one can have megabytes of data collected per day, if not more.

As stated before, this chapter focuses on the actual delivery of the service. So assuming that from a medical point of view, we have crafted the perfect solution and we still must take care that the service is highly scalable, robust, and cost of operations is as low as possible. It is essential that the patient is guided in using the devices, and how to deal with technical issues. There must be a contact person available to solve any problems with the equipment and so on and so forth. On top you have to enable a consistent quality management system that provides all reports that are required by the involved stakeholders.

It must be possible to reconfigure existing functions and enable further services and functions to the same patient; these might be provided by other service providers. Some shall be free of use; others have to be charged, either to the payer or the patient himself. This assembly of services must be designed comprehensively, and it must ensure that all regulatory, compliance, and billing issues are adequately managed. Last but not least, one must care about the life cycle of the product, this starts with the introduction to the market and ends with the planned exit under predefined conditions.

So in summary, we face a complex set of task including:

- Service assembly, design, market entry, and exit
- Patient education and training
- Service activation and configuration
- Management of service operations and patient problems
- Remote device management
- Logistics and repairs
- Quality management
- Billing and charging.

None of these have a primary medical meaning, but they have major implication on the quality of the delivered medical care and are mission critical issues from a telecommunications perspective.

A Brief Look into Evolution of Standards in Telecommunications

If one wants to create residential-oriented large-scale deployments of health services, it requires a robust technology infrastructure that addresses efficient design, development, deployment, operations, and billing of these services. This is where well-established capabilities of the telecommunications industry are very helpful to scale digital health services to have a population impact.

For example, consider a mobile network where a carrier is managing several millions of SIM cards attached to multiple services combined with a myriad of different contracts and pricings. The carrier maintains operations support systems; call centers for sales and support; billing systems and so on. Over the last decades, the telecommunications industry has managed to vastly improve cost efficiency while decreasing time to market for new service offerings.

The telecommunications industry has developed industry standards from its early days. But as the value propositions have shifted from technology to business service providers, the traditionally technology-oriented standards had to be supplemented by business- and process-oriented models. This evolution becomes evident when looking at the key important standards that have emerged over the last decade and the focus within these standards (Fig 7.1).

The first notable standard that was introducing the notion of a business view was the telecommunications management network (TMN). It started in 1985 and is a protocol model defined by ITU-T [1] for managing open systems in a communications network. The first TMN recommendation [2] was published in 1988, it was developed further until 1996 [3]. The TMN model consists of four layers.

Business Management. It performs functions related to business aspects, analyzes trends, and quality issues (e.g., Finance, HR).
Service Management. It performs functions for the handling of services in the network such as definition, administration, and charging of services [e.g., Order Handling, Service Licensing Agreements (SLAs)].
Network Management. It performs functions for distribution of network resources: configuration, control, and supervision of the network. (e.g., Planning, Maintenance, Statistics, Error recovery).
Element Management. It contains functions for the handling of individual network elements. This includes alarm management, handling of information, backup, logging, and maintenance of hardware and software.

From a top-down approach, each layer imposes requirements on the layer below; while from a bottom-up approach, each layer provides capabilities to the layer above.

The next step in evolution of telecommunications process models was the Telecommunications Operations Map, called TOM. The main development happened between 1995 and 1998 by the Telemanagement Forum [4]. By 1999, TOM was considered to be stable. TOM was using the TMN model as a foundation and added operations support and management for any communications service.

The key enhancement toward TMN was the introduction of the customer perspective. Instead of only looking at the internal management aspects of networks, the acknowledgment of customer needs was introduced into the modeling context.

The TOM process framework is independent of organization, services, and technology. It provides the framework for modeling end-to-end business processes from a top-down and customer-oriented standpoint.

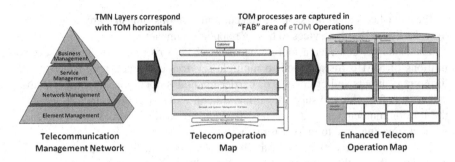

Fig. 7.1 The evolution of the network management standards shows the shift toward consideration of strategic and customer needs

The evolution continued in the year 2000 with the introduction of the enhanced Telecom Operation Map, called eTOM [5]. It has been adopted by the ITU-T as process standard ITU-T M.3050.x [6]. The eTOM is a broader framework and more complex than the TOM. It integrates e-business and internet opportunities while maintaining the top orientation of business processes. The eTOM further strengthens the customer driver approach since e-business has shifted markets from a supply orientation to a demand orientation or push versus pull. Most importantly is the introduction of the Strategy, Infrastructure, and Planning process domain (SIP). In this domain, the required processes for managing product life cycles over the layers from market to technology are defined. Today, eTOM is the most widely used and accepted standard for business processes in the telecommunications industry. The eTOM model describes the full scope of business processes required by a service provider and defines key elements and how they interact.

The eTOM Business Process Framework serves as the blueprint for process direction and the starting point for development and integration of Business and Operations Support System (BSS and OSS, respectively). The whole purpose of these processes and IT systems is that everything "works according to plan". As profit margins in telecommunications are extremely thin, it is paramount that these support processes and systems work at maximum cost efficiency.

A second major driver in telecommunications is customer experience. In times where most technologies can be provided by most providers in similar quality, the customer experience is a key differentiator for a provider. Today, the customers have one service center that they can call which will take care of all customer concerns. These may range from the inquiry about service availability and pricing, ordering of new services, management of customer problems, or questions on invoices. The TMForum Case Study handbook series provide good examples how carriers such as BT, Vodafone, Telefonica, Deutsche Telekom, Telstra, and many other companies achieved impressive efficiency and quality improvements by adopting standards like eTOM [7].

So in summary, there is a broad foundation at hand and it is highly recommended to explore the reuse of these frameworks for the efficient delivery of digital health services.

Some of the most obvious communalities are as follows:

- Management of large-scale deployment
- Serviceability of remote services and devices
- Management of customer interactions
- Management of access policies to data and functions
- Ensure service quality and availability
- Charging, billing, and invoicing
- Low cost of operations.

Utilizing these frameworks has some benefits from adopting best practices such as:

- Lower risk for failure due to end-to-end management view
- Lower cost of launch and operations of services
- Efficiency by reusing available processes and systems
- New value chains for telecommunication providers
- Clear separation for concerns.

Example for Application of the Concepts

At first hand, all this might look a bit abstract, and therefore, let us mirror this framework to a potential architecture for digital health service offerings (Fig. 7.2).

The core concept being adopted in this example is the separation of horizontal management domains. This concept enables the multi-party collaboration for joint service offerings. It creates one joint view of the service toward the patient; the roles and responsibilities of every involved participant can be clearly defined.

The horizontal tiers are a slight simplification of the TMN layers demonstrated above.

Product   All commercial aspects of the product are addressed here
Service   This layer includes the technical services that provide the product
Resource This layer includes logical and physical elements that are used in the provision of the service and product (e.g., mobile phone and monitoring app)

Looking at the example of the cardiovascular patient, a well-structured architecture model can now be the basis for one joint view of the service toward the patient and the roles and responsibilities of every involved participant.

By applying the structure of the above framework, one can define the monitoring service as business product based on technical services and resources/infrastructure. Every tier is managed within its own management domain; within this

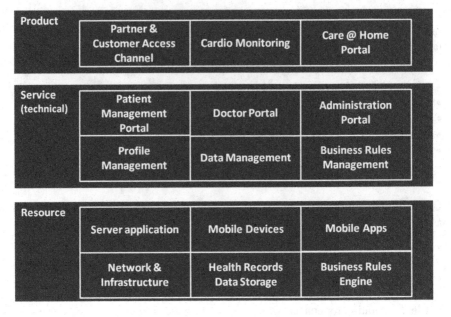

Fig. 7.2 The separation of commercial and technical aspects leads to high flexibility for designing new product offers

domain, you can define clear owners and handover points. This approach provides the global overview and management of all levels of detail at the same time.

Here, we provide an example for structuring a cardiovascular telemonitoring service.

The commercial product in this example is sold as B2B offering to insurance companies. The insurance company itself decides how to market this as B2C offering to its own residential clients. A similar principle you would find, for instance, with a mobile virtual network operator (MNVNO) that provides its own market products but does not own a network. The branding and access to the end customers (or rather patients) is provided and managed by the respective "reseller," in our case the insurance. The same product like cardiomonitoring might be offered by various insurances. All capabilities of a layer rely on the capabilities of the layers below. Therefore, another product such as "Care @ Home" may use a subset of the very same technical services and resources below.

Product: Cardiomonitoring

Description   This product is hosted by telco ACME and offered as resale product to insurances. It bundles all sub-services such as device delivery and activation, training for use of devices, call center for problem handling, medical assistance, alarm and attendance, medication reminders

Owner   ACME telco.

Service: Cardiomonitoring Portal

Description   Online portal for service ordering and activation, ordering of hard-
               ware, management of patient data records, access to patient health
               records, QM reports, etc.
Owner   ACME telco.

Service: On call nurse

Description   Call center with medical trained staff. Is available at configured
               times. Provides regular checkup call for patient
Owner   Medical Call center provider XYZ.

Service: Mobile nurse

Description   Mobile nursing provider. Nurses do regular visits to patient's home.
               In case of emergency, a nurse will be dispatched to the patient
Owner   Mobile nursing provider XYZ.

Service: Remote blood pressure data collection

Description   This service collects the data from the remote blood pressure
               devices and stores these as CDA records in a central storage
Owner   Device manufacturer ABC.

Resource: Remote blood pressure devices

Description   Mobile devices for the measurement of blood pressure
Owner   Device manufacturer ABC.

This architecture is now very powerful from a product design perspective. It allows adding more services and resources to the same product or defining new products on the available services and resources. You can define promotions, bundles, and so on. The key enabler is the strict separation between the customer/product and the technology layers.

Ultimately, the product specification is determined by the medical use. It is also the single point of truth when it comes to pricing. In other words, the product specification defines the requirements for all subsequent technical capabilities. The technical capabilities in turn offer the building blocks for new commercial product bundles. This allows you to clearly structure your roles and responsibilities throughout the product development process.

Two major benefits are the reusability of the technology services which drive down cost and risk of delivery and significantly improve time to market and profitability. This provides an overview of how telecommunications companies and digital service providers can utilize business and technology standards with the processes listed above to scale digital health services and offer these services at attractive price points. There is a lot of work that goes on in the background that patients and clinicians do not see.

Managing Multi-partner Cooperation

Having defined the management domains is one first important step. The next is to commonly structure the operational processes and handover points. This is essential since the operations of the digital services require the participation of multiple stakeholders. A common challenge of such multi-party cooperation is the lack of "the big picture." The natural consequences are that optimizations can only be created locally within the domain of a single party. This becomes even more challenging if you consider the profit loss responsibility of each single entity. Every organization optimizes its own profit margin but this rarely translates into better outcome for the patient.

To counteract these local optimizations, it requires global key performance indicators (KPIs). These are the basis for driving any change and optimization. For the sake of global quality management, one must be able to define strict service level agreements (SLA) and have the required data points at hand to enforce adequate reporting. But you can only define these KPIs and SLAs if you have some good understanding of the entire path of all activities related to the digital health service.

A domain management model is a good starting point for getting some overview. Detecon International has published in 2013 an end-to-end domain model that is based on TMForum Process Model (Fig. 7.3).

The domain model defines five management domains.

The patient-centric domain represents the patient view and interaction with eHealth. These processes start with the patient initiating the contact and end with the fulfillment of his/her need.

The health management domain represents the internally triggered patient view and interaction within the care provider. Processes include activities such as prevention and patient record history management.

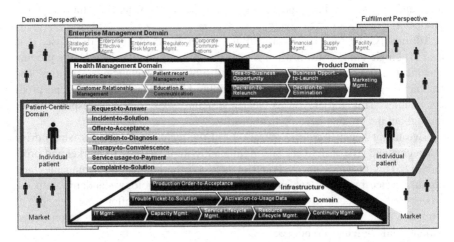

Fig. 7.3 The domain model provides a blueprint to design end 2 end processes for management of patient needs

The service domain represents the product and marketing view and interaction within eHealth. Processes include activities such as product lifecycle management (PLM), innovation management, and marketing management

The infrastructure domain represents the IT and infrastructure operations view and interaction within the company. Processes include activities such as order handling, trouble ticket management, and service lifecycle management.

The enterprise support domain represents the internal administrative view and interaction within the company. Processes include activities such as general management, HR management, and supply chain.

Since this domain model is build on top of the eTOM process model, it takes advantage of the more than 500 process building blocks that are already pre-defined. The process model itself is backed with a shared data and information model (SID), which is not further discussed here. The used standard models provide you a massive head start to define a solid end-to-end management view.

Of course, one must use this model with some caution since eTOM was developed for telecommunications. There is still some work to be done to carefully review applicability of every process step. First results look very promising however. A Detecon International study from 2011 [10] demonstrates quite a significant match of eTOM to health requirements (Fig. 7.4).

To get better hands on idea on how to use the domain model, let us use a process of the patient-centric domain to demonstrate the management of patient-triggered activities.

For instance, there must be some kind of enrollment process that is the initial trigger for a subscription of the patient. The **condition-to-diagnosis process** defines the activities starting with a (unspecific) health issue perceived by the patient to a sound diagnosis and recommendation of therapy.

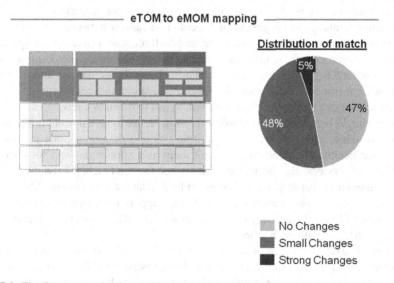

Fig. 7.4 The Detecon study shows that in particular the service and resource management related process definitions indicate a high degree of reusability

This process provides the blueprint to define how a patient might be enrolled into the program, e.g., who is authorized to enroll (the patient himself or just the doctor); what are the procedures, workflows, and rules for checking eligibility in terms of insurance cover and medical status (contraindications and comorbidities, insurance plan, etc.).

Key advantages of this process lead approach are completeness and reusability.

Imagine you have to adopt the same service for new regulatory requirements or you would like to launch a similar product. In this case, you are building on a sound and tested template. All this in turn translates back to lower cost and time for service launch and lower risk for failure.

Do not Reinvent, Be Clever, and Combine

Having outlined some well-established core concepts of telecommunications, we would like to close this chapter on joining this view with also widely adopted standards of the medical space.

Standards for telecommunications focus on managing large-scale operations of distributed digital services. They provide the basis for the design and management of all processes and systems to enable and support the service delivery. State of the art OSS and BSS systems and processes are content agnostic. So it does not really matter if a customer service center serves telephony or IP TV services even though the lower layers of networks and protocols may be vastly different.

So following this idea the medical payload of medical data and services becomes just another type of media content. Of course, we have to obey strict regulations for access to data, regulatory issues etc. But all these concerns also exist in the space of telecommunications. ITU-T provides a series of recommendations that address the requirements for management of telecommunications networks [8]. Standards for identity management, service quality, and fault management are building on top of these recommendations. Equipment and software vendors are providing software suites that are implementing these standards. These cover partner and customer management, product catalogues, for service activation and configuration, service assurance, service quality management, billing just to mention a few.

This should be another good reason to consider reuse to save upfront investments.

In our view, one can use the capabilities of telecommunications industry to frame the health data standards and treat them as a special payload for telecommunication services. Below we can visually see the relationship between key telecommunications capabilities and common health data standards (Fig. 7.5).

The service delivery capabilities enable the support systems and processes that are responsible for the delivery of the health services. Therefore, the standards harmonize perfectly with each other.

A good example is for instance HL7 [9]. The HL7 organization, which is accredited by the American National Standards Institute (ANSI), has the mission to develop standards for the healthcare industry worldwide. "Level 7" refers to the seventh level of the International Organization for Standardization (ISO) seven-layer

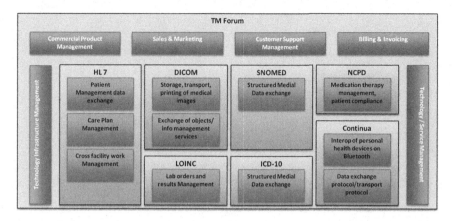

Fig. 7.5 Framework capabilities are framing health standard capabilities and enable efficient service creation and delivery

communications model for Open Systems Interconnection (OSI)—the application level. The underlying assumption is that all layers for ensuring the physical and logical transmission of data including error control etc. are provided by the OSI layers 1–6. The management of these layers is subject to the OSS/BSS standards of the telecommunications arena.

One expected outcome of such well-aligned management domains is that health professionals can focus on health payload while telecommunications professionals can focus on service delivery. The domain alignment provides the basis for efficient communication between the domain experts. A desirable consequence will be that next generation health services can be delivered faster, more secure, at better quality and at a lower cost point.

References

1. International Telecommunication Union. http://www.itu.int/net/ITU-T.
2. CCITT Blue Book. Recommendation M.30, principles for a telecommunications management network. vol. IV. Fascicle IV.1, Geneva; 1989.
3. CCITT. Recommendation M.3010, principles for a telecommunications management network. Geneva; 1996.
4. TeleManagement Forum, founded 1988. http://www.tmforum.org.
5. GB921. The Business Process Framework (eTOM). http://www.tmforum.org.
6. ITU-T Recommendation M.3050.x Series enhanced telecom operations map. 2006. http://www.itu.int/rec/T-REC-M.3050.1-200703-I/en.
7. TMF-Case Study-handbooks. www.tmforum.org.
8. ITU-T Recommendation M.3010 (2000). Principles for a telecommunications management network.
9. Health Level Seven International (HL7). http://www.hl7.org.
10. Detecon Study on transferability of eTOM to Healthcare. 2011. Detecon International GmbH.

Chapter 8
Smart Healthy Cities: A Case Study from Brazil in Public–Private Partnerships

Washington Tavares, Katia Galvane and Jody Ranck

Introduction: Why PPPs in Digital Health and Smart Cities?

Public–private partnerships have been growing in popularity over the past decade. From global health market failures for drugs and vaccines to major infrastructure-related investments, PPPs have become an important vehicle for both public and private value creation when normal market mechanisms fail to meet public needs. Increasingly, governments are attracted to PPP models in the context of a long-term financial crisis as a means to drive innovation or productivity without incurring as high levels of risk or debt. PwC estimates that BRIC and OECD countries will spend more than $68.1 trillion between 2010 and 2020 on non-infrastructure issues.[1] This level of expenditures will demand greater government efficiencies and means a growth in opportunities for private industry to partner in synergistic ways. The past history of healthcare sector PPPs was largely focused on infrastructure without much attention to technology, but we are now entering a new phase of healthcare PPPs focused on services. Digital health will be one of the focal points for redesigning healthcare systems for quality improvements at a

---

[1]Build and Beyond: The (r)evolution of healthcare PPPs. December 2011.

W. Tavares (✉) · K. Galvane
Tacira Technologies, São Paulo, Brazil
e-mail: wtavares@tacira.com

K. Galvane
e-mail: katia.galvane@tacira.com

J. Ranck
Strategy and Business Development, Ram Group, Washington, D.C., USA
e-mail: jody.ranck@ramgroup.com.sg

© Springer International Publishing Switzerland 2016
J. Ranck (ed.), *Disruptive Cooperation in Digital Health*,
DOI 10.1007/978-3-319-40980-1_8

lower cost. New incentives are slowly taking hold and will gradually move the incentives in healthcare away from the traditional "sickness" economy to a more prevention and wellness focus over the next decade. Another important area for PPPs is the growing business in smart cities which by definition, must be a public–private partnership. We will explore some of the emerging issues and innovations that are happening in Brazil and how they may help build critical frameworks for creating smart healthy cities in the future.

New digital health PPPs will demand new strategies and ways of thinking about innovation. National-level technology strategies are entering into a new era where investments in education and IT infrastructure fueled by more open approaches to innovation will be required to meet the demands of a more agile marketplace and more demanding patients and citizens. Open innovation requires skill sets in collaboration, managing social processes and platforms. We see this with the impact that social media is having in healthcare almost daily as even hospitals are developing social media strategies. PPPs can offer a means to share risk across both public and private sectors while offering a means to stimulate productivity and innovation in resource-constrained contexts. For many observers of public sector investments, PPPs offer a more strategic and entrepreneurial approach for government investments than many traditional, more bureaucratic approaches to investment. In some national contexts where privatization efforts have become controversial, PPPs when structured appropriately have offered a less controversial means for improving efficiencies in services while still maintaining public trust.[2] In the global health arena, a number of PPPs were launched in the late 1990s to address market failures for new drugs and vaccines for neglected diseases. Partnerships such as the Global Alliance (Global Alliance for Vaccines and Immunizations, formerly GAVI) brought together global health donors such as the World Bank and the World Health Organizations and private funding from the Bill and Melinda Gates Foundation to offer incentives and innovative financing mechanisms to incentivize private sector biopharmaceutical companies to develop new vaccines for diphtheria, tetanus, and pertussis to name a few.

In the digital health domain, we are seeing growing interest in the use of PPPs and cooperative business models to help transform health systems through adoption of new health information technologies, or digital health products and services. The telecommunications sector is eagerly embracing the idea of cooperative business models as they look at the complexity of healthcare systems and healthcare challenges. Globally, health systems are straining to provide higher quality care at a lower price point. Governments have the ability to shape markets for health IT as the largest consumer of health IT, but the nimbleness that the technology sector requires is rarely the strong suit of government. The consumer electronics industry is in the early days of making forays into the digital health arena, but the effects of how this industry operates are already being felt in healthcare.

---

[2]Kikeri, S. and J Nellis. 2004. "As Assessment of Privatization." The World Bank Research Observer, Vol 19, No. 1, Spring 2004.

Healthcare and medicine are accustomed to a more top-down, reductionist approach to services that has reached a turning point where the next generation of leaders and innovators will be those who can master more participatory, distributed, and localized types of services and approaches to care. This will be a market with much greater transparency in the past and PPPs will need to respond to these trends as well as address the regulatory cultures that are struggling to keep up with the rapid pace of technological change. Engagement with the public is going to be a key ingredient of success of both government and private sector healthcare innovations in the future, as we found in our work on best practices and case studies on successful efforts to "bend the cost curve" in healthcare globally.[3]

There is a great deal of risk in health IT from the perspective of entrepreneurs and private sector players. Physicians and the health sector in general have been slow adopters of new technologies. Health systems are some of the most complex sectors of the economy with many legacy systems that have created a large number of silos that often defy market rationalities. In the case of the USA, fragmentation of the healthcare system is exacerbated due to the unique history of the evolution of healthcare that has been employer-driven, dominated by a large number of small medical practices that make scaling up new technology systems a rather challenging endeavor. Even in developing country and middle-income markets such as Brazil, there is fragmentation due to the existence of both public and private sector markets for healthcare. One indicator of the complexity of the US healthcare system can be seen in a recent Institute of Medicine report that estimates the level of healthcare expenditures lost to inefficiencies and waste annually to reach over $750 billion.[4] There are dramatic costs associated with fragmentation and inefficiencies that also have an impact on health outcomes and patient safety. Health IT is expected to play a major role in addressing these challenges in the coming years as we have seen with the investment incentives in the HITECH Act. It is a well-known fact that sharing data across government agencies and private sector companies is a serious challenge for all parties involved. Recent developments with health standards such as HL7's Fast Healthcare Interoperability Resources (FHIR) standard may alleviate some of these challenges, but this will likely take several years more before there is a robust deployment globally across systems.

Transparency through open data and new accountability incentives that are driving adoption of health IT will make the effects of the data silos and lack of interoperability more visible in the coming years. The same holds true for urban planning where silos across the sectors that city must manage, from transportation to healthcare, result in less efficient services. To maintain economic competitiveness, countries and cities will need to cut waste and develop more nimble medical

---

[3]PwC, 2012. Healthcast: Global Best Practices in Bending the Cost Curve.

[4]Institute of Medicine, 2012, Best Care at Lower Cost. The Path to Continuously Learning Health Care in America. National Academies Press.

technology and urban planning sectors. These trends along with several of the trends we have identified from the PPP sector should help inform strategies and designs for PPPs. Some of the key drivers of PPPs that PwC has documented from their PPP practice area include the following[5]:

- Investment Need: A shift from assets to efficient operations. Growth in health-care expenditures due to aging societies and chronic diseases during a period of significant belt tightening provides an important incentives for governments to look to the private sector for efficiency gains in both healthcare and urban planning.
- Better Procurement: Shifting government's role from provider to regulator. With nearly two decades of PPP experience, a number of private organizations have developed the capacity to work with governments on PPPs and vice versa. There is also a need to bring both the public and private sectors into alignment to strengthen the overall system. PPPs are a proven vehicle to accomplish this.
- Access to Skills and Knowledge: Health PPPs require more than dealmakers. As healthcare PPPs move beyond infrastructure, they will require a more diverse array of experts and stakeholders. As they shift to a focus on improving health outcomes, they will be working more with networks and information technologies and seeking ways to overcome the silos and fragmentation that have hampered health systems to date. This is going to be a central facet for digital health PPPs.
- Service Capacity: Infrastructure PPPs have had a focus in the past on hospital beds which can further feed the perverse incentives in health systems that drive up costs. Emerging PPP models will seek to go beyond the models used in the past.

Challenges for PPPs

One of the most difficult technological and business challenges for healthcare systems has been the lack of interoperability of health IT services. It is not uncommon to find within a single hospital a scenario where the different IT systems used by different departments (laboratory, operations and financing, clinical, billing) are not interoperable. This is one of the problems that smart cities technologies work to resolve as well. This has implications for patient safety and the quality of care and has become an important dimension of "meaningful use" requirements for compliance with the government EHR incentive programs. A team of researchers at Harvard University that focuses on interoperability challenges across different sectors has identified several of the underlying elements of interoperability

---

[5]ibid.

that make building interoperable IT systems a challenge. In a recent book, *Interop: The Promise and Perils of Highly Connected Systems,* John Palfrey and Urs Glaser have mapped out the risks and dimensions of interoperability with some insights into the various roles that both government and the private sector can play. There are four major dimensions to interoperability that they have identified:

- Technological layer: hardware and computing systems
- Data layer: data from EMRs and other devices as well as standards used across the telecommunications and health systems
- Human layer: how human beings on each side of an exchange communicate and work together
- Institutional layer: the legal frameworks, internal processes, and rules that guide institutional behavior.

Palfrey and Glaser note that one of the most difficult challenges for interoperability in the healthcare sector has been the issue of different actors in the system having different meanings of interoperability depending on the context and technologies used. This is clearly an issue where governments through vehicles such as PPPs can use their convening power to bring a diverse system of stakeholders together and co-create the "rules of the road" that can satisfy both the business and regulatory requirements from which to build a sustainable technological and business framework that can have the scale and optimum level of interoperability to safeguard privacy and security standards as well as improve patient safety, health outcomes, and the continuity of care. When the market gets too far out in front of the "backend" issues of interoperability, reimbursement policies, and so on, we run the risk of contributing to fragmentation in the system and making the goal of better care at lower cost as a goal in the distant future. We will address the interoperability challenge in more detail later, but this is an obvious issue where PPPs could make an important contribution in the coming years. In the global health arena, there has been some activity in recent years to build PPP structures to address interoperability challenges in developing country markets such as the HI-PPP (Health Informatics-PPP) funded by PEPFAR that has focused on developing an enterprise architecture for national-level eHealth systems in Rwanda, Cambodia, Mozambique, and Zimbabwe.

Mobile network operators (MNOs) increasingly view the interoperability challenge as a business opportunity where they can leverage their strengths in networks, cloud computing, and enterprise-level data management capacity. PPPs in digital health and smart cities should also be aware of the dynamics of change in the telecommunications sector. Chetan Sharma has identified the dominant trends in the telecommunications sector that may also shape the engagement of MNOs in digital health in the coming years.[6] MNOs are facing a transition point or the

---

[6]Sharma, Chetan, 2012. Operator's Dilemma (And Opportunity): The 4th Wave. Mobile Future Forward Paper. http://www.chetansharma.com/OperatorsDilemmaFourthWave.htm.

fourth cycle in their maturation. The first waves involved voice and text messaging as their primary revenue sources. In the fourth wave, MNOs must find ways to eliminate costs and produce efficiencies while simultaneously driving innovation in data and applications for their consumers while fighting off competition from "over-the-top" competitors such as Facebook, Google, and Microsoft. These dynamics are fed by a growing market in the area of "digital lifestyle" solutions that include health and wellness. This has profound implications for business models and the way MNOs will operate in the future. The era of dumb pipes and a focus on an increasing number of smart devices (rapidly becoming commodities) is going to give way to offerings that focus more on smarter solutions, enterprise-level integration of data and devices. In other words, a New Service Economy for telecommunications.[7] MNOs are beginning to engage in more open innovation strategies that mark a departure from the past. The demands of the New Service Economy and those who see the new innovation landscape emerging recognize that new skills around cooperation and co-creation are going to be in higher demand. This will likely be a major trend that will influence the shape of emerging PPP practices at the intersection of health and telecommunications in the coming years. Yet healthcare still lacks serious platform approaches to services as we see in other sectors of the economy. When the health IT systems evolve to become more API-driven, we will likely see platforms that generate new business models the way that Apple, Facebook, Google, and Amazon have in healthcare. Ideally, this would make health services more patient-centric and enable greater liquidity of data.

New Service Economy, Digital Health, and PPPs

Digital health PPPs can certainly build on the lessons of PPPs past; however, there is also an opportunity to innovate in terms of strategies, platforms, and innovation approaches that a PPP nestled at the intersection of information technology and healthcare can aspire to in the coming years. Innovation in digital health will demand that we grasp the broader dynamics of the emerging digital economy and digital lifestyle offerings and understand how these may shape consumer engagement with prevention and healthcare in the coming years. Some deep thinking around the structural shifts that we are now undergoing in both sectors could be useful for plotting the path forward and identifying emerging opportunities. What both healthcare and telecommunications are now grappling with is a new technological revolution that will fundamentally shift business models and innovation strategies in the coming years. One view of the deeper transformation comes from

---

[7]See Jody Ranck, 2012, Mobile Operators and Digital Health. Mobihealthnews, 2012 Report.

the work of political economist John Zysman (UC Berkeley) and the other from the Italian philosopher of information, Luciano Floridi. PPPs that understand this transition and are designed to catalyze innovation in this context may be more successful in generating a willing pool of private sector suitors as well as offering opportunities for the public as co-creators and participants in design of new services. While the complexities of such partnerships are more challenging, novel designs may go a long way in generating political support as well as build on successful precedents that have been implemented in the open data space in recent years.

Zysman has spent much of the past decade studying the digital revolution and what it means for the overall economy and how governments and companies need to rethink innovation in the area of digital services. What we are now going through is an "algorithmic revolution" that is about the growing application of rule-based information technologies and tools to activities we label as services.[8] In contrast to the services of the past, the New Service Economy is the source of high value creation. Many services that were once performed by workers providing highly personal activities can now be performed through the use of sensors, mobiles, and other technologies requiring a different set of skilled workers to manage the technologies and often removed from the place where the services are provided. We see this happening slowly in telehealth and telemedicine with the use of outsourced radiologists, for example, who provide teleconsultations to health systems in the USA but from telemedicine centers in India. Furthermore, the algorithmic revolution often blurs the distinction between product and service. Think of how the iPod and iTunes worked in tandem to up-end the music industry. The iPod provides a channel or distribution point for access to the service, iTunes. General Motors makes money from its OnStar Service even when the platform for the service, the car, is declining.[9]

The algorithmic revolution has implications for how countries rethink national technology and innovation strategies. Zysman argues that the implications mean finding more nimble innovation processes and modular approaches to problem solving, finding innovative ways to manage increasingly fragmented knowledge, and balancing the flexibility of workforce management with adequate social supports. On the latter issue, he looks to Denmark where the flexibility of US companies and the social supports of France find a finer balance than either the USA or France. But the central dimension is the management of two key stacks of tools:

- The Data Network Stack
- The Service Tools Stack.

---

[8]John Zysman, 2006, The Fourth Service Transformation: The Algorithmic Revolution. http://brie.berkeley.edu/publications/wp171.pdf.

[9]ibid.

These two layers will be important for digital health PPPs going forward. Many organizations are currently focusing on a device such as the mobile. However, the range of sensors and technologies is growing and the technology ecosystem deployed in the management of chronic diseases and wellness, for example, may be very different three years from now. What is important to recognize is that data and services build around the devices are where value creation will happen. Since PPPs are generally long-term relationships, it will be important to have a somewhat agnostic framing of the technology that can encompass technological evolution but also not lose sight of the health data needs and economics of health data. The World Economic Forum has recognized the growing economic value of personal data so far as to proclaim personal data as a "New Asset Class".[10] Alongside the growing economic value of data, we find growing controversy over the uses of data by the private sector as well as new cultures of data sharing and data philanthropy. Therefore, the data network stack should be taken seriously as an area for investigation and significant PPP activity and innovation that could generate new products and services derived from data that may benefit under-served communities. This is an area of significant market failures at the moment but could also be sources of significant public and private value creation as we will explore later.

PPPs will need the foresight to play a role in these various transformations and identify the key leverage points where public–private cooperation can facilitate value creation for the public as well as contributing to a vibrant, competitive ecosystem in digital health. This is where the complexity of government strategies across sectors and divisions within government often become a roadblock to sectoral innovation strategies. The national broadband strategies of Japan and South Korea and how these efforts encountered numerous roadblocks to success when different pieces of broadband challenge fell under different ministries with diverse goals. PPP architects will need to map these roadblocks and have the ability to convene parties from across, not only the private sector, but different parts of government to form at least tacit consensus around the major barriers that could undermine long-term success of digital health PPPs. PPP managers could have an important role as facilitators and managers through the creation of trusted, neutral spaces along a variety of axes.

The cycle depicted below illustrates the need to rethink how governments in the New Service Economy will likely need to operate. While skeptics of government may view the challenge as overwhelming, there are already some examples of actually existing practices in US government ranging from the new Consumer Financial Protection Bureau to the Health Data Initiative of Health and Human Services that have created a precedent to build upon, and we will visit these later.

---

[10]World Economic Forum, 2011. Personal Data: The Emergence of a New Asset Class. http://www.weforum.org/reports/personal-data-emergence-new-asset-class.

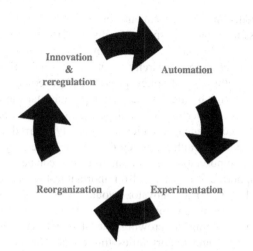

Innovation and Experimentation in the New Service Economy. *Source* John Zysman (2006). Services, Networks, and Competition: Creating Value in a Digital Era.

In digital health, the lack of clarity around the future regulatory environment is frequently cited as a roadblock to investment and innovation. While PPPs have limitations on the role of the private sector in discussions of regulatory issues, there are clearly opportunities for cooperation around coordination of the multitude of government agencies that can help shape the environment for digital health. One of the difficult challenges for policy-makers is creating a regulatory environment that remains current with the rate of technological change. In some countries, telehealth and telemedicine could technically be illegal due to the technology policies created in the 1980s–early 1990s that are still on the books and pre-date the technologies that are actually in place. Cloud computing offers an interesting case study in this regard when servers for a particular cloud computing application are geographically located outside of the country of origin of use of the service. Data privacy and security regulations pre-dating cloud computing services can occasionally render the service as a privacy violation in some national contexts.

A final note on the transformation of health and data comes from Luciano Floridi, the philosopher of information, who has been studying the effect of the information revolution on healthcare and medicine. Floridi observes that we are now in the Fourth Technological Revolution (Copernicus, Darwin, and Freud launched the first three) inspired by the development of the computer by Alan Turing. The impact this has had on healthcare is that digital health technologies are rendering the body more more transparent (e.g., MRIs render the body into a digital format), shareable (we can share the data from our trackers on platforms like Patientslikeme.com), and more democratized (the web and information about health and wellness are making access to health and medical knowledge more widespread and usable as tools by a wider variety of people). Information is increasingly embedded in our environments, or infospheres, as Floridi terms it. It is almost meaningless to empirically speak of a divide between the online and offline world(s) as information becomes embedded in our environments. We are moving from an era of informational scarcity to an era of information overabundance which will require a rethinking of policy, privacy, and governance. This means that for digital health and digital cities, we are dealing with a far more engaged set of users with vastly more powerful tools and platforms at their fingertips, literally. We are increasingly seeing engaged patients, frequently referred to as "e-Patients", asserting their voices into health IT policy debates in some very important ways. They now have very important online communities that can be useful platforms for policy creation, support. e-Patients are also important test beds and user communities for digital health tools, and innovators would be foolish to neglect their value and voices in the creation of new innovation ecosystems.

PwC has been researching the growing role of social media in healthcare and some of the challenges and opportunities this creates for healthcare organizations in our social media "likes" healthcare (http://pwchealth.com/cgi-local/hregister.cgi/reg/health-care-social-media-report.pdf) report. There are lessons here even for PPPs given the new environment for consumers of healthcare in a more social media-driven world. Consumers are expecting more transparency and faster responsiveness to their issues. This creates substantial challenges for even leading edge private sector healthcare businesses, but the challenges are even greater for government. There are also opportunities to leverage the platforms for research, ideas for greater patient engagement, and marketing of efforts. These will be more pertinent to PPPs of the future than we have seen in the past.

Goals of Digital Health PPPs

PwC's Health Research Institute has taken a global perspective on health sector PPPs and generated substantial insights on where trends in the PPP domain will go in the coming years. In *Build and Beyond: The (r)evolution of healthcare PPPs* they have presented an analysis of the various models and the transition to more service-oriented PPPs in the coming years. Healthcare PPPs since the 1990s have focused predominantly on healthcare infrastructure such as hospitals and medical facilities or product develops partnerships for drugs, vaccines, and diagnostics. With the emphasis now of system efficiencies, prevention, and chronic diseases, the opportunity space for digital health PPPs is growing. In global health, there have been a few early PPPs to emerge in the area of mHealth:

- SMS for Life[11] is a PPP that involves the Tanzania government, Novartis, CDC, and academic partners to address the problem of stockouts and supply chain management for anti-malaria drugs

---

[11]http://malaria.novartis.com/innovation/sms-for-life/index.shtml.

- Health Informatics PPP (HI-PPP)[12] is a global partnership to develop health information systems in low-resource settings with HIV prevalence rates. It is funded by PEPFAR and has several NGO/social business partners including INSTEDD, Jembi, Regenstreif Institute, WHO, Public Health Informatics Institute and focuses on developing enterprise architecture frameworks for inter-operable systems
- Maternal Alliance for Mobile Action (MAMA)[13]: an mHealth PPP focusing on maternal health formed by Johnson and Johnson, USAID, mHealth Alliance, and Baby Center.

These early examples of digital health PPPs in the global health context have largely focused on the use of SMS and rather simple tools that can be deployed readily in low-resource contexts with the exception of the HI-PPP endeavor that is a much more complex task centered on both front-end and back-end technology development that can strengthen entire health systems. The HI-PPP is also more politically complex due to the focus on "country ownership" of the process when local skills to manage complex health informatics systems are in short supply. The tension point here also highlights a possible PPP opportunity for partnerships that can build the health informatics knowledge and expertise for health systems globally. The shortage of health informaticians may only grow in the coming years as the private sector need for data scientists grows and pulls individuals out of the public sector where wages are lower.

From our review of PPP projects globally, we have identified a number of insights for both government and the private sector as they build new partnerships.

For Governments:

- Establishing a national framework for PPPs that includes standardized processes, risk management, and contracting expertise is important for developing professional discipline as well as the flexibility that can enable PPPs to succeed in the long run
- Investment in skill teams that can deliver results. Many governments will be able to leverage expertise from past PPPs to apply these skills to next-generation service-oriented PPPs
- Flexibility is a key element of success particularly with rapidly changing technologies
- Entrepreneurial approach and thinking: This involves transparency, business plans execution, and staying in tune with consumer preferences.

For Business:

- Focus on lowering costs: measuring outputs of the PPP and the value for money and efficiencies created

---

[12]HI-PPP.org.

[13]http://www.babycenter.com/mama.

- Share the risk according to competencies: Government can transfer risks that are better managed by the private sector such as in areas of new technology development and professional development
- Accept fair margins: responsible behavior that support competitive and efficient capital structures while government should also acknowledge fair margins that can support a sustainable long-term partnership
- Reassess what information is proprietary and what should be published. Transparency on metrics can help build public support for PPPs. Resistance to PPPs often comes from public views that private firms are the primary beneficiaries of PPPs. Demonstrating increased access to care and quality of care and/ or cost savings will generate support.

We will now turn to a case study of smart cities that actually responds to some of the issues outlined by PwC above in this introduction to PPPs. Telefonica Vivo and ISPM, both in Brasil, are piloting an approach to smart cities that aims to fill in some of the gaps with existing smart cities programs and create new efficiencies and more effective approaches to building smart cities in a modular fashion.

Smart Cities and Cooperation Case Study in Brazil: Telefonica Brasil and ISPM Cooperate with Local Governments

Smart cities represent one of the best use cases for cooperative business models given the public–private partnership model that is inherently part of the operating business model. Smart cities are based on the premise that networking technologies, sensors, and data analytics can provide citizens of cities and city managers the ability to dramatically improve services and facilitate the overcoming of data and communications silos that characterize most city planning departments. The market for smart cities technologies is expected to reach \$400 billion by 2020.[14] As the internet of things and big data continue to grow, the range of services and technologies that can be utilized by cities will only grow. This is why it is important at the current conjuncture to put into the place the basic standards and frameworks that can enable more efficient and effective development of smart cities initiatives. This is where smart cities need to learn from the mistakes of many health systems around the problem of interoperability that plagues most health systems attempting to appropriate digital health technologies for system-wide improvements. The lack of use of standards and common frameworks to guide both city planners and technology companies can impede growth in this area. For this reason, Telefonica and ISPM have initiated a cooperative project to build the frameworks for creating a modular approach and business model for smart cities through a pilot program in

---

[14]Pike Research, http://www.greenbiz.com/news/2013/03/06/growth-smart-cities
https://www.gov.uk/government/news/new-initiative-to-support-40-billion-smart-cities-in-the-uk.

Brazil. This chapter will provide an outline of the approach that we are currently deploying in a small city in Brazil, Águas de São Pedro.

Smart Cities and Health

The most popular smart cities technologies tend to be those associated with transportation and smart grid technologies. These use sensors and geospatial systems to monitor traffic flows in real time and provide data on traffic patterns to city planners. But the actual range of smart cities initiatives is far more vast with applications in everything from education to smart grids, economic and financial systems, and smart buildings. Healthcare is also an important city service in most cities and urban planners must manage a broad range of factors that are linked to health outcomes. In the 1980s, the World Health Organization launched the healthy cities and communities initiative that combined urban planning with public health in order to think pragmatically about a more holistic approach to health planning. Under this vision, traffice and physical infrastructure are important inputs for producing better health outcomes. Brazil was at the forefront in many ways for the healthy cities movement in cities such as Porto Alegre who utilized participatory budgeting initiatives that became some of the most innovative approaches to building more inclusive cities and in the process gained important insights into how residents "used" the city and their infrastructural needs and offered a mechanism for citizens to play a central role in improving public health outcomes in a democratic manner. Today, we have an opportunity to use tools such as open data initiatives, technologies, and healthy cities initiatives in a coherent way to improve the public's health. However, interoperability across these sectors remains a major challenge. A quick look at the complexity of this challenge also highlights the importance of building a framework to address the underlying architecture, standards, and business models in order to build platforms capable of meeting the health needs of cities.

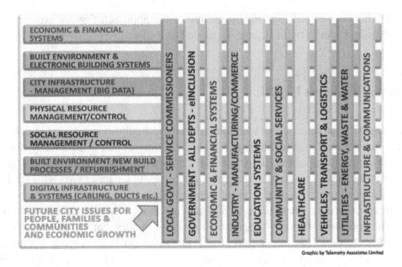

Graphic by Telemetry Associates Limited

Case Study: Águas de São Pedro: The First 100 % Digital City in Brazil

Telefônica Vivo initiated an important pilot project in Águas de São Pedro, a small coastal city known for its tourism industry, and a population that swells from 4000 to several fold higher during tourism season (but this program involves a number of other companies including ISPM, Ericsson, Fundação Vanzolini, Grupo Bem, DataNext, Informar Saúde, Gol Grupo, Huawei, and _Onthespot). This means transportation issues can become a major problem during certain parts of the year. The goal is to prepare a new type of infrastructure for the city to enhance digital services for the population, businesses, and city managers using both data and voice enabled services initially. What this means in a context like Águas de São Pedro is a major transition from a network that was 100 % copper cable to fiber optics and a move away from one centralized telefonics center to handle all of the services to a multiservice cluster of 5 networked centers to serve the needs of the population. The initial investment for this segment of the project costs nearly $US 900,000 and was needed to significantly upgrade the quality of digital services that the city could provide to citizens. But the investment offers a payback for local businesses who can now use the much faster bandwidth to offer more rapid, higher quality services that can take advantage of streaming, gaming, file backup and storage, etc.

The initial infrastructure upgrade will then form the foundation for building a new generation of connected services: digital education, tourism, eHealth, and municipal management. In the digital health arena, this means better access to medical records and care plans as well as telehealth services that can connect physicians and patients to specialty care centers, the ability to manage public health campaigns for issues such as dengue fever that are a serious problem during rainy seasons, general health education campaigns, and the development of a new Health Portal for the general public to access health information from public health agencies.

The broader initiative will enable the city to better monitor energy use and find efficiencies across the city. An important area is transportation, particularly during high tourist season where monitoring traffic flows will enable better mobility and monitoring of air quality levels throughout the city. Other applications include public safety initiatives that can monitor lighting in cities and breakdowns in infrastructure that could cause public safety issues such as crime rates to increase where lighting declines. An education initiative that will involve smartphones and tablets is also being developed.

One of the challenges that vendors currently have with city governments is the lack of standards and common frameworks that both vendors and city planners can use to prioritize and plan smart cities as well as implement programs in a modular manner that does not lead to silos in services and data usage. The telecommunications industry (see Chap. 7) has a set of standards for business practices that we cover in our chapter on the telecommunications approach to developing digital health services, can be extremely useful in developing the building blocks for piloting and scaling up digital services across the verticals that smart cities focus on. The first step that we will be implementing is research that leads to the creation of profiles of different cities by digital service *needs*. Modular components for digital services can then be developed that match the set of needs that various cities have and they can pilot individual services initially while adding on new layers of services in a coherent interoperable manner.

Some of the initial experiences with smart cities globally have demonstrated that purely top-down, technocentric approaches often encounter resistance or lack of engagement by the users of the city, that is, citizens. A number of observers of the first generation of smart cities have noted that participatory approaches will be a key ingredient for future success so we will be looking at the use of open data and civic hackathons where students, citizens, programmers-at-large have an opportunity to identify gaps in services and then co-create services with the smart cities initiatives. Telefônica Vivo has extensive experience in the digital health and broader digital services space with these types of programs via the "Campus Parties" and business accelerators/incubators sponsored at various universities and cities to catalyze further innovation on the platforms created by Telefônica Brasil.

Chapter 9
eHealth Policy in LMICS: National Frontiers, Global Challenges

Ticia Gerber

Introduction

The World Health Organization (WHO) defines eHealth as the use of ICT for health.[1] eHealth involves the application of tools such as telemedicine, health information systems, mobile and medical devices, e-learning platforms, and decision support systems. eHealth is employed to improve the delivery of health services and to support better health and health systems throughout the world. eHealth projects continue to expand globally. Initiatives are being implemented in more than 100 nations[2] with an eHealth marketplace estimated at $96 billion and growing.[3] Collectively, these developments present a timely opportunity to address persistent health system challenges, support the march toward achieving the health-related Millennium Development Goals (MDGS), deliver critical services across the continuum of care, and to promote progress on larger health systems issues such as more equitable resource allocation and improved governance and leadership.

---

[1]World Health Organization. *eHealth resolution* (Resolution WHA 58.28). Geneva: 58th World Health Assembly Resolutions, Decisions and Annexes List; 16–25 May 2005; Available from URL: http://apps.who.int/gb/or/e/e_wha58r1.html; pp. 108–110.

[2]World Health Organization, *Atlas: eHealth country profiles*. Geneva: The Global Observatory for eHealth; 2011; p. 7.

[3]Boston Consulting Group, *Understanding the eHealth Market*, Bellagio Making the eHealth Connection Conference, 2008, p. 3.

T. Gerber (✉)
Partnerships and Policy, HL7, Washington, D.C., USA
e-mail: gerbergroup2@gmail.com

© Springer International Publishing Switzerland 2016
J. Ranck (ed.), *Disruptive Cooperation in Digital Health*,
DOI 10.1007/978-3-319-40980-1_9

As the use of eHealth expands, a number of groups, including policymakers, international organizations, donors, funders, academicians, and implementers, are calling for increased agreement on the eHealth principles, standards, tools, and policies used by different countries and more alignment of eHealth projects and programs with national health priorities. For example, the report on the Global Strategy for Women's and Children's Health calls for, among other things, support of country-led health plans, and innovative, efficient approaches to integrated health service delivery.

References to increased agreement on eHealth are included in WHO resolutions,[4,5] efforts of the Global Health Initiative (GHI)[6] and Calls to Action by the H8,[7] PARIS21,[8] the Rockefeller Foundation's Making the eHealth Connection collective[9], and the Global Health Information Forum.[10] Expert coalitions, particularly in Africa and Asia, have progressed on devising technical design and standardization guidelines for eHealth, open architecture coordination, and best practices in eHealth implementation in low-resource settings. Despite these declarations and well-intentioned efforts, the challenge of effective public policy that supports such infrastructure looms large, particularly in developing countries where health care and system inequities can be more pronounced.

During the last decade, I have investigated and worked to improve eHealth policy process, resources, and coordination in LMICs through field work, education, and global diplomacy. This chapter outlines my critical synthesized learnings for the benefit of LMIC health ministers and for the larger field of global eHealth stakeholders including donors, government decision-makers, researchers, and

---

[4]World Health Organization. *Strengthening health information systems* (Resolution WHA 60.27). Geneva: 60th World Health Assembly Resolutions, Decisions and Annexes List; 14–23 May 2007; Available from URL: http://apps.who.int/gb/or/e/e_ss1-wha60r1.html; pp. 100–102.

[5]World Health Organization. *eHealth resolution* (Resolution WHA 58.28). Geneva: 58th World Health Assembly Resolutions, Decisions and Annexes List; 16–25 May 2005; Available from URL: http://apps.who.int/gb/or/e/e_wha58r1.html; pp. 108–110.

[6]U.S. Global Health Initiative. *Global Health Initiative at a Glance*. Available from URL: http://www.ghi.gov/about/index.htm.

[7]Chan M, Kazatchkine M, Lob-Levyt J, Obaid T, Schweizer J, et al. *A call for action on health data from eight global health agencies: meeting the demand for results and accountability*. PLoS Med 2010; 7(1): e1000223. Available from URL: doi:10.1371/journal.pmed.1000223.

[8]Participants of the PARIS21 2009 Consortium meeting. *Dakar declaration on the development of statistics*. Paris: PARIS21; November 2009; Available from URL: http://www.oecd.org/docum ent/48/0,3343,en_21571361_41755755_41760432_1_1_1,00.html.

[9]Rockefeller Foundation. Making the eHealth Connection, Sign on signatories [Internet]. New York (NY):Rockefeller Foundation; [cited 2012 Jan 8]. Available from URL: http://ehealth-connection.org/ehealthpetition/212.

[10]Participants of the Prince Mahidol Award Conference (PMAC) 2010 Global Health Information Forum. *Call to action: global health information forum*. Bangkok: PMAC; January 2010; Available from URL: http://www.pmaconference.mahidol.ac.th/index.php?option=com_content &view=article&id=201%3Acall-to-action-final&catid=966%3A2010-conference&Itemid=152.

other experts. The insights from this work will prove helpful in building future cooperative initiatives in many developing countries.

LMIC eHealth Policy—National Considerations

Policy is a set of statements, directives, regulations, laws, and judicial interpretations that direct and manage the life cycle of an issue.[11] Studies conducted by WHO, the Health Metrics Network, and others have revealed that policy is among the weakest components of country eHealth and health information systems. This failing is a growing tension point in low- and middle-income countries (LMICS) where eHealth projects and programs continue to expand. A recent study found eHealth projects or programs operating in 58 LMICs on the continents of Africa, Asia, Europe, and the Americas. Countries most frequently cited as eHealth hotspots are as follows: Kenya, India, Tanzania, Rwanda, South Africa, Peru, Vietnam, Thailand, the Philippines, Indonesia, and China. While eHealth project reach is significant, so are budgets. LMIC eHealth projects have an average dedicated budget expenditure of $900,000 USD per annum.[12] This suggests a powerful and wide scope for health technology initiatives with an acute need for effective tools and policies.

LMIC countries that introduce and implement eHealth generally encounter one or more of the following policy development issues:

1. Drafting a high-level eHealth policy roadmap;
2. Translating high-level eHealth policy into language for national legislation;
3. Updating an already established eHealth policy; or
4. Facilitating cross-border eHealth policy collaboration with other countries.

One of the first helpful steps to undertake in the policy development process is to review relevant information in global, consensus-based principles, declarations and calls to action related to eHealth. Examples of such documents include declarations by the H8 (http://www.plosmedicine.org/article/info%3Adoi%2F10.1371%2 Fjournal.pmed.1000223),[13] PARIS21 (http://www.paris21.org/sites/default/files/ DDDS-en.pdf),[14] participants of the 2010 Global Health Information Forum

---

[11]Richard J, et al. Telehealth policy—looking for global complementarity. *Telemed Telecare* 2002;8 (Supp 3).

[12]Gerber, T and Seebreghts C. *Aligning eHealth Initiatives for Results*, p. 3. Study Results Available from URL:
http://www.globalhit.net/IDRC-Results/.

[13]Chan M, Kazatchkine M, Lob-Levyt J, Obaid T, Schweizer J, et al. A call for action on health data from eight global health agencies: meeting the demand for results and accountability. *PLoS Med 2010*; 7(1): e1000223. Available from URL: doi:10.1371/journal.pmed.1000223.

[14]Participants of the PARIS21 2009 Consortium meeting. *Dakar declaration on the development of statistics*. Paris: PARIS21; November 2009; Available from URL: http://www.paris21.org/ sites/default/files/DDDS-en.pdf.

(http://www.pmaconference.mahidol.ac.th/index.php?option=com_content&view
=article&id=201%3Acall-to-action-final&catid=966%3A2010-conference&Ite
mid=152.),[15] and the 2007 World Health Assembly Resolution 60.27 (http://apps.
who.int/gb/ebwha/pdf_files/WHASSA_WHA60-Rec1/E/cover-intro-60-en.pdf) on
Strengthening Health Information Systems.[16]

A second helpful step in the eHealth policy development process is to review
and better understand how other countries have addressed with these issues. The
World Health Organization's Global Observatory for eHealth (http://www.who.
int/goe/data/en/) is an excellent place to start for insight on these issues as is the
eHealth Resource Section of the Asian eHealth Network (http://www.aehin.
org/Resources/eHealth.aspx) and the ICT Toolkit for Women's and Children's
Health(http://www.who.int/pmnch/knowledge/publications/ict/en/).

And finally, as national LMIC ministers and others plan the introduction and/
or expanded implementation of health information systems, a multitude of in-
depth policy questions must be considered. The list of queries below can serve as
a launching pad for such a discussion. Key questions are in the areas of: (1) data
stewardship; (2) governance and accountability; (3) workforce training and capacity building; (4) architecture and interoperability; and (5) financing.

Key LMIC eHealth Policy Questions

Data Stewardship

1. What are appropriate eHealth information-sharing and data policies?
2. What policies are required for effective eHealth information transfer and
   reporting between regional, district, and national facilities? Will policy require
   personal identifiers?
3. Will policy mandate the appointment of a Chief Data Officer at the national
   and/or district levels for effective eHealth information management?
4. Will policy mandate the establishment of an eHealth data repository? If so,
   what are the appropriate requirements to govern such repositories?

Governance and Accountability

1. What key policies strengthen the government's institutional capacity to conduct
   eHealth policy planning, management, regulation and enforcement?

---

[15]Participants of the Prince Mahidol Award Conference (PMAC) 2010 Global Health Information
Forum. *Call to action: global health information forum.* Bangkok:PMAC; January 2010;
Available from URL: http://www.pmaconference.mahidol.ac.th/index.php?option=com_content
&view=article&id=201%3Acall-to-action-final&catid=966%3A2010-conference&Itemid=152.

[16]World Health Organization. *Strengthening health information systems.* Geneva: 60th World
Health Assembly Resolution List; 2007; Available from URL: http://apps.who.int/gb/ebwha/pdf_
files/WHASSA_WHA60-Rec1/E/cover-intro-60-en.pdf.

2. How can diverse governmental parties responsible for eHealth policy be effectively coordinated and managed? Is a multi-stakeholder committee required?
3. How can non-governmental actors and private sector players be encouraged to participate in eHealth policy development and implementation? Will policy incentivize or mandate such participation?
4. How can eHealth data be collected in compatible formats and submitted regularly to relevant authorities using harmonized reporting?
5. How can eHealth policy integrate and align with national health strategic and reform plans, relevant international mandates, and donor program requirements?

Workforce Training and Capacity Building (Human Resources)

1. What policies support adequate eHealth staffing levels, effective staff training, and retention related to HIS? What lessons can be learned from capacity-building policies and efforts in areas of health care?
2. How can policy support an expansion of in-country legislative specialists and/or increased technical assistance to draft or update eHealth policy?
3. What eHealth policy information can be offered on a free, open access basis to increase knowledge transfer?

Architecture and Interoperability

1. What are the key elements of policy that will support integrated eHealth (e.g., system integration and better interoperability)?
2. What policies can be put forward at the country and global level to ensure increased participation in the standards development process and more cost-effective standards access?
3. How can the international standards harmonization process and policy support eHealth strengthening?

Financing

1. What type of donor collaboration and cooperation can support eHealth development nationally and across borders?
2. What funding and business models lead to eHealth sustainability and how can they be supported and incentivized through policy?
3. How can collaborative public and private sector eHealth funding models be encouraged?
4. How can informative and regularly updated documents about eHealth progress be created for diverse stakeholder such as ministers, system users, healthcare providers, patients, and the media?

Global Issues

1. How can eHealth policy priorities be integrated into the health agendas of global institutions and moved forward?
2. How can effective eHealth policy across borders be achieved?

Emerging LMIC eHealth Policy Gaps

As efforts advance to gather information about existing eHealth policy in LMICs, key questions, roadblocks, and clear policy gaps have emerged. Overarching challenges identified through in-country and global policy stakeholder engagement to date include things such as:

- **The difficulty and time-intensive nature of crafting meaningful and detailed legislation from high-level policy statements;**
- **Policy Teeth**—"Policy" can have very different meaning in LMIC context, for example, policy can be an outline of a plan that has not even been considered by the legislature.
- **Locating existing regulations related to eHealth which are nested in diverse, often antiquated laws, and governed by numerous ministers.** Common national laws to be examined in eHealth policy formulation include but are not limited to: national health strategic and reform plans, sanitary codes, national statistical acts, marriage, birth and death registries, privacy and security practices, freedom of information acts, digital signature requirements, hospital and healthcare provider reimbursement, e-government, and health systems strengthening initiatives. Policy alignment with requirements from donors and international bodies must also be considered.
- **Achieving effective stakeholder engagement and coordination on eHealth policy within the government and between the public and private sectors in fragmented systems with multi-sectoral responsibility is difficult.** National ministers that may be involved in national eHealth policy can include Ministers of Health, HIS, Public Health and Social Welfare, Sanitation, Labor, Finance, Telecommunications, ICT or eHealth, Justice, Immigration, and Education. The National Statistics Office and experts in charge of such issues as e-government will also be consulted.
- **A shortage of qualified policy staff and experts at the national level and a revolving door of consultants;**
- **Inadequate education on standards and interoperability issues and lack of a standard collaborative to fill the gap;**
- **Addressing tricky and controversial data access issues;**
- **District and local solutions at play**—LMICs have more locally driven and customizable strategies: e.g., open source tools and community and non-traditional health workers.
- **Maintaining eHealth project financing and sustainability in an environment of competing priorities and political instability.**
- **Donor Alignment is an issue**—Multiple donors mean multiple policy alignment, evaluation, and reporting issues.
- **The Overlay of Global Goals and Institutions**—Policymakers look to MDGs, WHO, and regional bodies for guidance and policy alignment. eHealth often must been seen and dealt with through the prism of major global health issues such as health system strengthening, health equity, universal health coverage,

civil registration and vital statistics, and/or capacity building or large-scale infrastructure reform. Constantly realigning eHealth with the global health flavor of the month can dilute, muddy, and obscure health technology programs, implementation, and results.

LMIC eHealth Policy: A New Model

Clear and workable policy is a key anchor for successful LMIC eHealth implementation. However, to move forward in this area, attention must be focused on:

- Increased sharing of eHealth implementation experiences;
- More dialogue between eHealth movements (eHealth, mHealth and health information systems);
- Bolstering available resources on policy best practices;
- Supporting the development of country-level laws and growing advocacy related to eHealth in LMICs;
- Finding new and cost-efficient ways to address challenging policy gaps;
- Building reuse considerations and interoperability principles into eHealth;
- Forming a collaborative of national eHealth Stakeholder Councils;
- Conceiving new project funding models less tied to entrenched money sources and issue agendas;
- Informing donor thinking and giving, as well as larger global health policy discussions.

In pursuit of these goals, my recent strategic work has been to develop a framework for a new, iterative, and resource-rich eHealth policy model that empowers LMIC health ministers and includes the following on a regional and global scale.

Policy resources and activity	Description
Policy guides	A summary of existing notable activities national-level eHealth policy, an analysis of gaps that should be addressed and a guide for countries drafting or updating eHealth policy
Expert group discussions	Expert multi-stakeholder groups that discuss technical, legal, organizational, and policy issues in eHealth, leveraging global or regional meetings, and on-line discussion forums
eHealth legislative templates	Develop ready-to-use legislative templates that will guide countries in drafting and introducing eHealth policies
Resource center	Create a systematically updated center will contain eHealth policy resources and an online collaborating space to aid users
International policy resolution	Promote an official and actionable eHealth policy resolution could be taken up by global or regional bodies
Rapid response teams	Form flexible teams of noted technical, organizational, and policy experts that can be quickly deployed based on country or regional need

Important work continues on developing components of this model and seeking significant and collaborative funding for its deployment.

Conclusion

The provision of LMIC eHealth policy tools is crucial at this time when the UN Millennium Development Goals deadline is close at hand and many countries are moving toward health technology implementation. eHealth fundamentally supports more equitable, empowering, and sustainable health systems. And, policy can be a very powerful tool in achieving these objectives. As United Nations Secretary General Ban Ki-Moon states, "the right policies and actions, backed by adequate funding and strong political commitment, can yield results."[17]

---

[17]Moon, Ban Ki. *The millennium development goals report 2009* (Foreword Remarks). New York: The United Nations; 2009; Available from URL: http://www.un.org/millenniumgoals/pdf/MDG_Report_2009_ENG.pdf.

Chapter 10
Managing Cooperation for Information Security and Privacy in Health Care: A German Case Study

Cem Sentürk

What Is Information Security?

With the increasing data volume and digitalization in the society, the meaning of data privacy is an important issue. But what does it mean, when service providers try to protect data flows? It is important to create high-quality data, to securely store the data, to communicate the meaning of data, and finally, to use data for the strategic goals of an organization. On the one hand, data privacy is seen as a protection of misuse in the data processing which describes the structural and organized converting of databases, mostly used as a foundation for statistics in the scientific and economic area. Another important aspect, which has to be guaranteed through data privacy, is to guarantee individuals' privacy. Moreover, ownership and control of data is central. This right is a part of general privacy law but is also derived from the European Convention on Human Rights that says that everyone has the right to a private and family life. Service providers have to guarantee security, especially the privacy of their customers (patients). Because of this, information security is of growing interest and a priority in the telecommunications sector. In Fig. 10.1, we can see how it relates to the overall security picture.

IT security and privacy describe all of the technical arrangements of hardware and software which are necessary for the accessibility, integrity, and especially the maintenance of patient relevant data. Data security, on the other side covers the generic areas. They are composed by organizational, technical, and employee related sectors that are necessary for the correct processing of data. Data integrity is responsible for the storage, change, and integrated communication of data and is a link between the major columns of data privacy and security. The second link is built by data confidentiality. Its task is the protection against unauthorized

C. Sentürk (✉)
Detecon International GmbH, Cologne, Germany
e-mail: cem.sentuerk@detecon.com

© Springer International Publishing Switzerland 2016
J. Ranck (ed.), *Disruptive Cooperation in Digital Health*,
DOI 10.1007/978-3-319-40980-1_10

Fig. 10.1 Information
security framework (*Source*
Own research)

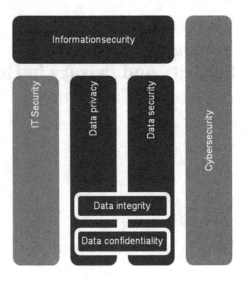

access to information. These definitions can be summarized by the umbrella term information security. Across from that definition, the concept of cybersecurity can be found. It describes the process of actions undertaken by the service providers to protect internally stored data from the outside world. With the presence of the Internet, this area has grown in importance. Naturally, data privacy and data security are in every industry matters that are treated with highest priority. It is especially important to protect personal-related data in the medical sector, to store data securely, and to maintain confidentiality and privacy. All of this means the health sector has a complicated challenge due to the strict privacy and security regulations and the need for maintaining the trust of patients and providers.

What is the Importance of Data Security in Digital Health?

Health enterprises must balance the need to reduce costs while increasing efficiencies and quality of care, all the while maintaining data security and privacy. Privacy standards and the legal obligation to store records are important to assure that medical data are only communicated to authorized medical providers. The exchange of data and the connected documentation of patient related data are extremely important to guarantee quality of care and seamlessness of care across providers. Healthcare data that are stored in databases offer the possibility. Handling data also carries risks such as exposure to hacking and cybersecurity threats. Hackers may manipulate software or, in the worse case get access to personal data and misuse them. Therefore, information security is a mission critical function. There are existing restrictions, such as information security for every party in the healthcare industry, but each of these pressure groups has its own goals, conceptions, and positioning.

How and Where Is It Relevant?

In the further enrollment of this chapter, information security will be discussed from the point of view of the three major parties of the public health sector. The focus is going to be on the patient, the provider, and the payer or insurer.

Patient

Trust is a vital form of social capital for healthcare institutions. Patient privacy and security building in the relationship with patients. One of the important dimensions of trust in a healthcare setting is consent management. It regulates which heath information from a patient is passed to the different providers and insurance companies. Furthermore, it enables patients to take part in e-health initiatives and to establish common frameworks to regulate who has, in any given context, access to a patient's data and the manner in which the data are passed from one provider to another along the continuum of care.

Provider

Providers have to offer an optimal medical treatment. They have also to take care of the confidential treatment of the generated data with the help of security systems. Here it is important to pay attention to the physical security of the documents. An additional security issue that requires appropriate hardware and software. This happens through lost or stolen data because of a lacking use of modern security technique. With the help of well-coordinated and secured IT systems, a consistent data transfer can be enabled through optimized processes. The organization must ensure that data transfers can happen without unauthorized personnel having access to the data. Data must also be anonymized and encrypted to ensure data integrity throughout the data flow.

Payers (Health Insurers)

Insurers are interested in controlling and forecasting medical costs therefore they require data regarding treatments so they can optimize care. Nevertheless, it is not always obvious which data they have access to. For the payers, it is important to have access to relevant data and to track billing and payments. It is important for insurers to assess the reimbursement and efficacy of treatments.

In this first section, we highlighted how information security is a major concern in the digital service economy and maintaining data security and integrity is central to the delivery of quality digital services. The following section will illustrate a simplified framework that can be used for building new services that meet the requirements for data privacy. How could a methodology for the implementation of information security look like?

Developing controls that are used to manage services across a number of data privacy and security domains are where we begin building our framework. These must cover the areas of data privacy, data confidentiality, data security, and data integrity as well as information security. In the telecommunications sector, there are numerous functional procedures that are already in use that provide guidance on delivery and monitoring of services. A given procedure is considered comprehensive and complete if it receives the designation "Data Privacy & Data Security Assessment" (DPDSA procedure). This designation guarantees a well-structured approach which has been followed in all of the sub-components of the data security and privacy protocols.

The information security level can be determined by categorizing a piece of data or process by project complexity and required safety and data privacy at the beginning of a projects' development. Therefore, it is focused on all systems and platforms, which are required to be constantly updated or newly set up. Furthermore, the DPDSA procedure enables an integrated process for data security and data privacy that builds upon the main component of the product and system development process. In this manner, multiple or identical information (redundancy) can be avoided and ensure that a better survey can be assured. This procedure offers the advantage of being applicable for any IT and NT systems, irrespective of size, complexity, and location of such a system. Optimized project support in combination with an appropriate safety level guarantees higher transparency during (ongoing) projects. After a successful categorization, a compendium consisting of all relevant client and provider data will be generated. It serves as a guideline for further actions and the documentation of project relevant security data. The final step consists of summarizing the projects' data and confirmation of the provider's approach.[1]

It is of particular importance that the provider is able to implement the following steps:

1. After the successful categorization of the project, the decision has to be made, whether the demand for supervision by designated specialists in terms of data and IT security is needed. Projects with a higher category are supervised by specialists/technical experts.
2. To enable a structured workflow during the project, it is important to update all systems that have been modified or newly set up as well as identifying the responsible employees. As a result, all relevant information is allocated in a central database that enables a structured and centralized process.
3. To meet the time targets, a smooth communication has to be assured between the parties. If because of the projects complexity, data privacy or IT specialists are deployed, it is especially important to take in consideration that a response concerning the project can require time. Therefore, documents relating to the specialists topics have to be handed in time.
4. During the whole process, it is highly important to coordinate the tasks and common actions of the parties involved and to preserve communication.
5. Under a steady documentation of the progress, the project can be continued after the control of the collected information from the specialist side.

---

[1]Source: Own research and development. In the context of various realized projects, a standard methodology or process model for implementation of information security was created.

Fig. 10.2 Overview and assessment of existing frameworks in relation to health care and information security (*Source* Author's own research)

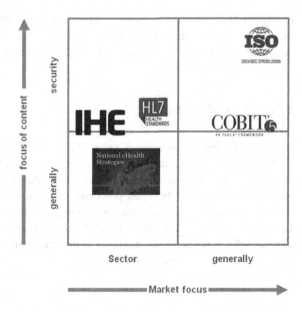

6. Regarding the later implemented security and data privacy requirements, it is extremely important to have a precise communication with suppliers and developers.

What Already Exists as a Best Practice?

There are different methods that can be used to protect information security. They differ mainly by their thematic focus. On the one hand, they are specified according to whether information security measures are treated exclusively or integrative. Another approach is based on whether they are to serve general or industry-specific requirements. When selecting a suitable framework, the question should focus on whether the central aim is the comprehensive protection of the information infrastructure or whether specific IT issues are at play and offer only a supporting role in the implementation of strategic security issues. In Fig. 10.2, important frameworks are shown and the following text will explain the main standards in more detail.

What Is ISO/IEC 270xx-Series?

The ISO/IEC 270xx series is a set of standards for information security whose content focus lies on the implementation and operation of information security management systems. A complete-implemented system covers the entire information security process of a company and serves as a framework for the central administration and the efficient management of a company.

What Is COBIT5?

Published by the Information Systems Audit and Control Association (ISACA)[2] COBIT Framework (Control Objectives for Information and Related Technology) is known as the international framework for IT governance. Here the approach is an end-to-end view of business processes of a company and the management of information and communication technologies. It focuses on the analysis of IT-related added value and business integration across the organization. Contextually, it is one of the frameworks that maps only in certain areas, with non-industry aspects of information security.

What Is HL7?

Health Level 7 (HL7) is a collection of international standards for the exchange of data between the information systems of various healthcare organizations. Since it is a communications standard for medical data in HL7, the topics of information security and privacy are of central interest. The transferred patient data must be protected from unauthorized access, loss, or forgery any time. The need for secure data handling is highlighted by a series of publications on information security, IT security, and data protection.

The Standard Guide for EDI (HL7) Communication Security,[3] for example, describes measures to ensure the confidentiality, integrity, and availability of patient data. In addition, the Health Level Seven Security Services Framework[4] supports in implementing comprehensive protection measures. By a very clear explanation also clarifies employees without explicit training in the field of information security, why the careful handling of patient data is necessary, what dangers lurk when dealing with information technology, and what measures they minimize errors.

---

[2]http://www.isaca.org.

[3]http://www.hl7.de/documentcenter/public/wg/secure/Hl7coms5.doc.

[4]http://www.hl7.org/documentcenter/public_temp_3D4771E9-1C23-BA17-0CC70F-C0FB041A00/wg/secure/HL7_Sec.html.

What Is IHE?

The Integrating the Healthcare Enterprise (IHE)[5] is an association of producers and users of information systems in the health sector with the aim to standardize the interoperability between IT systems. To support the implementation of best practices, IHE formulated use cases, identifies relevant standards (such as HL7), and develops technical guidelines (profiles), with which manufacturers can implement and test their products. In Germany, IHE is also supported by the German Radiological Society[6] and the Association of Healthcare IT.[7] Contextually, IHE as well as HL7 belong to a framework that has only an indirect relation to information security, but a direct relationship with the sector.

Information security and privacy are addressed in the IHE publications in different contexts and levels of detail. Depending on the type of profile physical security, processes or organizational aspects of information systems are in the foreground. The implementation of security measures is carried out by the publication of policies. In addition, each profile should contain the Security Considerations section. The content of this chapter is not a holistic safety assessment, but they will be considered only as aspects that are significant for the interoperability of the profile. To ensure an overarching protection of the information infrastructure, other frameworks should be used.

What Is the National e-health Strategy?

The National e-health Strategy is an initiative of the World Health Organization (WHO)[8] and the International Telecommunication Union (ITU).[9] It is a framework for developing national e-health vision, action plans, and monitoring model. Its implementation is planned by the participating governments. The strategy describes information security and privacy as an aspect of national e-health strategies and identifies them besides coding standards and data presentation standards as a key e-health enabler. An action plan includes publications of policies for information security and privacy as security and interoperability. The handling of patient data in the appropriate manner contributes to improving security and awareness of the implementing institutions.

---

[5]http://www.ihe.net.
[6]http://www.drg.de.
[7]http://www.bvitg.de.
[8]http://www.who.int.
[9]http://www.itu.int.

What Is Behind the Case Study:
Diabetes Prevention Portal

We will provide a concrete example of the use of information security profiles through the example of a diabetes prevention platform. The diabetes prevention portal provides a solution for the improvement of personal lifestyles for those affected by the disease. The general idea is to encourage more exercise and a healthier diet in the daily routines of patients with the monitoring support by personal coaches specifically instructed for this purpose.

This solution consists of mobile devices and an Internet portal. The blood sugar level and the exercises are measured at regular intervals and kept in a secure online diary. The diabetes patient is the only one having access to his data, but he can give access to these data to persons of trust like family members or the personal. The advantage of this portal is that the patient can talk at regular intervals with his personal coach regarding the monitoring of his or her lifestyle regimen and the determination of the next goals. In addition, the patient possesses the possibility to join a community of diabetics where he can exchange his experiences and information with others. This fosters motivation and can foster a sense of well-being. The diabetic benefits from the diabetes prevention portal, since he is better informed and monitored by the coaches and can exchange his experiences and fears with the community where she can receive peer support and encouragement. Hopefully, the anxieties of managing the condition can be reduced through coaching and peer support. Due to the ongoing information and monitoring by the coach, the deterioration of the diabetes or health status can be prevented by acting on early signals of non-compliance. A significant advantage of the diabetes prevention portal is that it can be put on the market quickly as an extended service to the existing services of the health insurance company.

The Concept

The patient enrolls with the portal, signs on to the program, and monitors daily lifestyle and health activities which are shared with a coach. In the event of a complication that cannot be handled by the coach, he can always resort to a doctor or hospital for support. The coach is in charge of setting-up the daily plan and of tailoring it to the individual patient. Therefore, the personal coach needs access to the recorded health data of the diabetic.

The completeness of the data is the prerequisite for the continuing therapy. A major challenge is to reach a consistent structure and accuracy of the data during the processing and communication between the different systems. Patients may use a variety of devices or apps. Another very important issue is to guarantee that only the designated persons or caregivers get access to the data and authorizations for access can be restricted by the patient. Therefore, solid access control and permission regimes are required meeting the expectations of the patients and the clinical staff which has led to a number of difficulties in the past. Privacy and data security are important assets but they should not hinder the data flow to the doctors. The challenge is to find a common basis for the data exchange. This will be of major importance for a successful implementation of the electronic health card in Germany.

The third party involved in running the diabetes prevention portal is the payor, i.e., the health insurance companies. They are in charge of controlling the costs and the training of personal coaches in order to ensure a constant therapy level. The ongoing training of the coaches enhances the odds that the health conditions of the patients will improve. For the payers, the diabetes prevention portal has the advantage that due to the better education and engagement of the diabetics and the close monitoring of risk of follow-up costs due to the long-term complications of heart disease, stroke, kidney failure, foot ulcers, and damage to the eyes will be lowered. When the patient feels treated well by the diabetes prevention portal program, this gives the payor a competitive edge over the other health insurance companies and improves retention.

The Program Sequence
The whole process starts with a message sent to the patient by e-mail, in which the key elements are explained. This includes the assessment of why the patient fits into the program, the start of the coaching, and the shipping of the hardware. The participant can at any time transfer the data collected by him to the diabetes prevention portal and thus enables the monitoring. The collected data will be illustrated in graphics and tables, and then explained by the coach. The communication with the patient takes place at regular, short intervals. The current status and future goals will be discussed and the coach gives guidance in order that these goals can be achieved. The communication between the patient and the coach is made possible by a news service.

The Participant
It is important for the patient to be able to use the provided devices correctly. The devices are recording the health parameters like blood sugar and the activities of the participant. These data should be transferred at regular intervals to the server to make a constant control possible. This allows the ability to correlate irregularities of the blood sugar with the activities in order to demonstrate the interaction to the patient. Meetings between the coach and the participants will be logged. In addition, the exchange of experiences among participants will be enabled via forums.

The Coach
The task of the coach is to have a good status overview of the participants assigned to him. The preparation of a patient interview requires a comprehensive view on

the patient with the help of the data diaries and the consideration of information from his superior. After a successful call, the key points have to be documented. The superior is responsible for the constant training and development of the coaches. At the end of each month, it is important to document in a report, what steps concerning the training of coaches have taken place and to what extent the objectives have been achieved.

In addition to the superior of the coach, there is also a medical supervisor. He grants approval for an applicant to participate in the diabetes prevention portal program. He also supports the coach with medical knowledge in the direct coaching and with the preparation of patient appointments in case of ambiguities or complications. Another field is to advise the coaches and to make an assessment on the achieved targets.[10]

What Can We Expect in the Future?

What Are the Challenges?

As outlined in the previous chapters, the challenges of data safety and security are raising with growing complexity of the portals.

It is advisable to not just rely on theoretical approaches but also address the practical questions that arise from the daily operations of such a portal. One aspect is to consider the rights and obligations of the service providers and other stakeholders concerning the access and use of private patient data.

There are also gray areas that are in need of careful analysis to understand better the pros and cons of different approaches and their relationships and dependencies. Different types of information and their relationship to each other have to be governed by different levels of security.

It is a logical consequence that the effort for security management measures grows with complexity. Security management efforts create significant cost and the bearing of this cost must be clarified as part of every provider model's service design. Costs can be spread across or covered by the patient, the provider, the payer/insurance company, or a government entity. As we will lay out in the next section, mixed models promise to be a successful approach to address this.[11]

---

[10]Source: Excerpt from a successfully completed project.

[11]Source: Own research.

What Are the Benefits for the Patient and the Perceived Real Threads?

The table below lists pro and con factors concerning data safety and security that will be elaborated upon further in this chapter.

Pro	Contra
Personalized treatment plans	Insurance can exclude patient from certain insurance programs/coverage
Anonymized or pseudonymized EHR data can also improve the efficiency and effectiveness of clinical research	Through connecting healthcare providers a rising complexity of security infrastructure
Reduce the risk of medical and prescription errors	Creation of "transparent" patient
Integrated infrastructure can make data available globally. Doctors can treat patients outside their country of residence	Sensible data can be accessed online by hackers any time

The "transparent" patient is a disturbing reality and a major benefit at the same time. The full availability of a patient's medical records history is necessary to provide the best care and avoid medical errors. This becomes even more relevant if a patient is abroad and on different time zones.

In the area of prevention or for dosage adjustment of medication during therapies, the additional data is a significant factor to improve quality, reduce cost, and improve patient outcomes. In case of emergencies, it is valuable for a hospital to have access to information on allergies, medication taken, and chronic diseases. This shortens decision times for choice of right procedures and improves quality of care.

The security frameworks of systems and underlying databases have to be carefully audited to ensure full compliance to all requirements for data safety and security. They also must provide a well thought balance between required patient benefit and associated threads.[12]

What Are the Opportunities?

This chapter outlines the areas of opportunity that could not be addressed without adequately design security standards.

One of the most important opportunities is a global, fully integrated system landscape. One prerequisite is the enforcement of the same level of security

---

[12]Source: Own research.

similar to what we find in online banking. One distinct difference, however, is that data abuse in the case of health may have a lot wider impact than in the field of banking. Such abuse has the potential to severely impact a person's reputation, leading to loss of job and social status.

The separation of patient health data records across multiple databases is a viable strategy. Patient identification is handled by one system whereas the medical records management is done elsewhere. A common key enables the correlation between the data sets. But this concept comes at a high cost for capital expenditure and operations.

Services such as social patient driven communities (health 2.0) enable the exchange between patients. Here patients can share experiences, motivate each other, discuss problems, and receive advise in a moderated but anonymous environment. The prerequisite to enable such solutions at a large scale with integration between multiple service providers is the overarching security policies and their reliable enforcement by organization and technology. They have to provide a good balance between sharing data and protecting the patient's data privacy.

These are just a few examples on potential and danger of online solutions. As technology is advancing and scale of systems becomes bigger, the requirements for security are getting more complex as well.

Chapter 11
Crowdsourcing Cooperation for Better Clinical Outcomes

Osama Alshaykh

Introduction

Article 25 of the Universal Declaration of Human Rights [9] establishes that all of us are entitled to medical care. This is easier said than done, especially when combined with the dominant justice and equity theme of the declaration. We may disagree if equity of medical care is realistic; however, most of us agree that it is a worthy goal. In this paper, I will present a new platform that facilitates cooperation in the sharing of medical knowledge that can address health equity challenges.

To illustrate the complexity of providing equity in medical care, imagine twins born in a poor community. A well-to-do couple in Boston adopts one child while the other child remains in the orphanage. Let us assume due to their genetic makeup, both have diabetes. Equity of care means both twins should have the same life expectancy. Dr. Paul Farmer [8] eloquently discussed equity and its importance for our global health and prosperity.

Urban communities are very diverse in terms of ethnicity, age, and income. They are made up of people from different backgrounds. Statistically, to improve care of such communities, we need to provide care that reflects the ethnic diversity of a community; otherwise, we will unintentionally neglect providing equitable care to people who paid for it and expect it. To do this properly, our medical research and practices should cover all races and genetic backgrounds and not only that of the majority of well-developed communities.

O. Alshaykh (✉)
nxtec Corporation and Boston University, Boston, USA
e-mail: osama@nxtec-corp.com

To achieve better care, we need to share information, knowledge, and practices. We also need to work together to solve local problems with global resources. That is, to solve an Ebola outbreak in West Africa, we need the knowledge of medical doctors in other parts of the world who have valuable expertise in that area who can work to complement local resources.

Connectivity and the Internet made the world smaller. Most of the world is connected (e.g., According to GSMA [3], as of 2015, half of the world has a mobile connection growing to 60 % in 2020). More importantly, 45 % of the developing world population is connected). People now exchange ideas, information, and work on projects regardless if they are in the same physical location or not. This leads to a new important tool: crowdsourcing.

According to the Merriam-Webster dictionary, crowdsourcing is "the practice of obtaining needed services, ideas, or content by soliciting contributions from a large group of people and especially from the online community rather than from traditional employees or suppliers." In a sense, it is brainstorming with experts with different backgrounds and experiences to solve a problem.

Crowdsourcing can be more powerful than traditional research, opinion polling, and one-on-one consultation. When you read an article, you are limited by your interpretation of the concept. Reading other interpretations and asking people for their opinion broadens the understanding and opens more solution avenues. Imagine medical professionals from different backgrounds discussing a certain outbreak, the collective knowledge of this group will be much larger than that of one consultant or specialist.

Crowdsourcing and open collaboration is an important tool to bridge the geographic knowledge gap. Specialists and experts from any part of the world will be able to provide specific opinions and help people that do not have access to such knowledge. Moreover, the specialists and experts will be exposed to more information by working on more problems and more scenarios.

Connectivity + crowdsourcing are fundamental and important tools to provide equity of care and improve the overall care of everyone. This chapter will discuss using crowdsourcing for healthcare.

Medical Information and Knowledge Is Special

Medical information deals with our physical and mental quality of life. In many cases, medical information could be the difference between life-and-death situations. For this reason, we should deal with medical knowledge and information differently. Discussing the treatment of a cancer patient is different that discussing how to restart a stalled car. The discussion forums are not for everyone. Moreover, few opinions matter even among doctors. For example, the opinion of a cardiologist about how to treat prostate cancer is not as relevant when compared to that of an oncologist.

Medical knowledge is built upon clinical cases. Access to the knowledge means applying it to scenarios that include people, symptoms, and environment. Moreover, the scenario is not always static. What this means is sharing medical knowledge is providing accessibility to a complex set of tools and actions that depend on changing scenarios.

The other important fact about medical knowledge is that its application may differ from one patient to another. The diagnosis may depend on social practices that the patient may not be comfortable sharing in public, or on genetic makeup that the patient would rather keep secret. At least 70 % of health outcomes are related to social, environmental, and behavioral issues that are managed outside of the clinic. This personal nature of the medical discussion demands significant attention to privacy and security.

Sources of Medical Knowledge

Practicing medicine depends on knowledge acquired by evidence (evidence-based medicine) and experience [1]. Both are very important. Evidence-based medicine provides information and knowledge based on carefully conducted experiments by researchers and experts. It is typically adopted and confirmed by prestigious medical board organizations. Medical experience is important because medicine is personal. Thus, the knowledge acquired by a clinician is important because they know firsthand what works best under certain circumstances.

Any medical information or collaboration tool must draw from these important sources. Moreover to succeed, such tools must:

- Be for everyone involved in the care of a patient and reviewed by medical experts. This includes direct feedback from the patient as her/his own advocate.
- Guarantee security and privacy.
- Embrace the dynamic nature of clinical encounters. Clinical discussions are not a typical question/answer sessions. They involve monitoring, follow-up, and multi-disciplinary opinions as well as coordination with a care management team for high-risk patients.

Collaboration and crowdsourcing are very important tools to communicate medical knowledge and improve it. If we are successful in building a viral application for medical professionals like Facebook, we can communicate state-of-the-art medical knowledge efficiently. Moreover, doctors can collaborate together to advance knowledge and exchange information, thus improving the overall knowledge of everyone.

Collaboration and Crowdsourcing in Healthcare

The main objectives of crowdsourcing in healthcare are:

- To provide access to specialists, i.e., medical professionals with special expertise and knowledge.
- To get fast conclusions on clinical cases based on expert-crowd-collective knowledge.

Applying crowdsourcing solutions to healthcare is not straightforward. There are special constraints in healthcare that need to be addressed in any solution, in particular:

- Privacy of patients and their information.
- Validity of the results.
- Legal and moral responsibility of the advices and contributors.

In the last couple of years, new types of healthcare applications have emerged that try to utilize medical doctors to provide expertise. The main categories of those applications are:

- Public expert question and answer applications: User post questions in a public forum and forum participants comment, advice, and suggest solutions. Typically in such applications, there are two kinds of participants: general audience and verified experts. Only experts with verified credentials can contribute. Everyone else are just readers of the interaction. Examples of such applications include Fig. 11.1 and CrowdMed.
- Public patient–doctor question and answer forums. Such applications provide a forum for the general public to ask doctors. Doctors can interact and provide answers. There are a large number of such applications including HealthTap, Sermo, and First Derm. The main problem of such applications is that many clinical cases require more interaction with the doctor than just posing a question. Moreover, patients may come to the wrong conclusion.
- Data Forums and centers. These are important forums where researchers post depersonalized data that other researchers can analyze and use in their research. Typically, results are published in peer-reviewed research conferences and journals. The interactions are delayed and not immediate.

Most of existing crowdsourcing healthcare applications focus on depersonalized clinical cases. Patients typically are presented with "Terms of Service" that are drafted to protect the application provider, the forum and their advisors. The "Terms of service" typically make it clear that the patient should consult her/his physician, who has the final say for that patient's care. Although these applications advance collaboration between doctors, their impact will be limited, mainly for the following reasons:

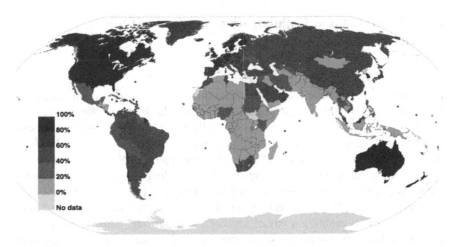

Fig. 11.1 Internet users as percentage of country population (from Odgen [7]; Jeff Ogden's own work, based on figures from the Wikipedia list of countries by number of Internet users article in the English Wikipedia, which is in turn based on figures from the International Telecommunications Union (ITU) for 2010 (updated to use figures for 2012 on 28 June 2013). http://en.wikipedia.org/wiki/Global_Internet_usage#mediaviewer/File:InternetPenetrationWorldMap.svg)

- Question and answer forums do not easily provide a vehicle for clinical case update, questioning, and medical test and care follow-up. The discussions are done in a spontanenous manner and it is the responsibility of the expert provider to connect the threads.
- Public discussions may have legal risks, resulting in many experts refraining from participating.
- The business models of such applications are under scrutiny. To elaborate, free applications claim that they will sustain their business by either advertisement or by sponsoring questions. The advertisers and sponsors are typically pharmaceutical companies, thus some may argue that this creates a conflict of interest. This is more concerning when the application providers pay for expert opinions, which is typically done to increase user base and market the application.

A new paradigm of crowdsourcing application is emerging. Such applications focus on building "virtual clinics," where medical professionals form a virtual clinic to discuss and solve medical cases. The main differentiator is that the discussion is private and not open to the public. This will make it easier to satisfy HIPAA and other privacy requirements allowing for more access to information and follow-up.

It is important to differentiate between this new category of applications and electronic medical records (EMR). An EMR system focuses on documenting a case. It does not focus on exchanging opinions and exploring diagnoses. The private forum provides this functionality. Examples of such applications include Tabeeb.

Crowdsourcing and Collaboration Are Access Tools for Knowledge and Expertise

Medical doctors are the center, brain, and heart of any healthcare system. Doctors, nurses, practitioners, medical assistants, and insurance companies must be aligned and in full communication to provide the best care for the patient. Access to medical doctors with special skills is key to providing the highest-quality care. We need cardiologists to diagnose and treat heart patients. We need oncologists to diagnose, treat, and care for cancer patients. Nurses and assistants administer the treatment and the specialist's knowledge is essential to providing quality care. Moreover, the role of nurses has evolved so much that they are becoming the responsible for primary care and in many cases chronic disease care.

Technology is enabling a virtual approach to healthcare, democratizing medical knowledge so that access to knowledge can be distributed and effectively used by more skilled healthcare professionals beyond doctors physically located with the patient.

Insurance companies can benefit from virtual healthcare by utilizing the best medical advice via crowdsourcing experts in their sphere of influence. Hospitals and clinics can financially benefit by providing experts advice to customers outside their geographic areas.

State-of-the-art medical information comes from different sources: bioscience research, clinical research, clinical practices and experiments, colleagues, healthcare data, and patients. It is important for us to provide tools that are integrated into clinical workflows for physicians to learn, interact, and share information while knowing that the source is trustworthy and the communication is secure.

It is also important to provide doctors with a platform or forum where they can ask questions and give opinions without the fear that this will impact their careers, and create legal risks. They need to be experts and students at the same time. Social media services, such as Facebook and Twitter, drafted Terms of Use policies that protect the company, not the users. For medical crowdsourcing, we need to encourage experts to participate by promoting their knowledge and legally protecting them from any backlash. We need new terms of service language for doctors and patients.

To summarize:

- Medical doctors are the heart of healthcare.
- Medical information can come from many sources. However, the credibility of the source is critical.
- Clinical decisions involve a significant number of factors.
- Healthcare systems have different constraints than other fields.

I will now provide a discussion for each of these four points.

Modeling Crowdsourcing and Collaboration Based on Typical Medical Interactions

Medical doctors' interaction with each other consists of:

- Person-to-person consultation. This could be a specialist asking the primary care physician for more information, a primary care physician confirming a diagnosis with a specialist or a doctor asking for advice. It is currently done via phone calls, emails, or private chats. It is limited to people who you know.
- Group discussions. This is when doctors and other medical professionals discuss a case together. They use collective knowledge to diagnose and create a care plan. It is currently done in-person.
- Medical community discussions. This is where people share experiences and research. It is currently done via journals and medical conferences.

To develop a comprehensive environment that can take medical professional interactions to the next level, we need a platform that includes:

- Expert-crowdsourcing tools, and
- Comprehensive media communications.

Merriam-Webster dictionary [6] defines crowdsourcing as *"the practice of obtaining needed services, ideas, or content by soliciting contributions from a large group of people and especially from the online community rather than from traditional employees or suppliers."* According to Merriam-Webster dictionary, the first use of the term was in 2006. When we add "expert," we restrict the online community to a group who has verifiable knowledge of the topic at hand. This is an important distinction because it is important that medical information and opinion shared be verifiable and come from a person of knowledge. The information shared will impact quality of life and in certain cases, it is a life-and-death decision.

   In an expert-crowdsourcing framework, doctors can exchange ideas and solve clinical cases together. In Tabeeb, a doctor posts a clinical case. The differences between a clinical case in Tabeeb and a social media post are:

- Clinical case information can be categorized in a clinical helpful way for doctors, e.g., history of the patient, symptoms, medication, tests including imaging, and diagnosis hypotheses. A social media post is a picture, video, or text. It is not comprehensive.
- Clinical cases are living entities. That is, the doctor who authored the case can always provide updates for the clinical case with progress or more information. The progress of a clinical case is an important differentiator from just a regular social media post. It provides doctors with a tool to experiment, update, and communicate in a way that resembles what they do on a daily basis.

- Media commenting and communications tools. It is important for doctors to interact together using pictures and videos. Sharing medical images is not enough. Doctors need to comment on pictures, draw on them and express their point of view visually. If we take this to next level, it means interaction between doctors by mimicking what they do with online tools, e.g., whiteboarding on images and annotation of videos and pictures with their voice.

Crowdsourcing enables interesting, informative, and meaningful discussions. If we combine the discussion with expert reviews, we can provide doctors with medical practice recommendations. For example, if three doctors are discussing a cardiac clinical case, the outcome of their discussion can be compared and combined with other ongoing clinical discussions via recommendation and filtering engines. The combination can be edited and reviewed by a panel of experts and promoted to become a practice recommendation. In this new era of expert crowdsourcing, this will expedite how medical practice recommendations are created and communicated.

Expert crowdsourcing can also benefit from online diagnostic tools. Borrowing from the banking industry, where models of different investment and spending habits are created, clinical discussions can also benefit from programmable views of clinical cases.

Appropriate Use Criteria (AUC) are very important for medical practice. AUC specify recommendations and procedures to perform based on evidence and expert opinion [1, 10]. AUC have been computerized. The next important leap for AUC is to utilize natural language processing (NLP) techniques and extract information from a clinical case and provide recommendation to the doctors involved in the discussion. This is the next step for Tabeeb, where it will provide such tools.

State-of-the-Art Tools to Provide Equity Access to Knowledge

Practicing medicine means staying current with a vast amount of biological, medical, sociological, and behavioral knowledge to keep patients healthy. Physician training, despite being quite rigorous, has omitted much of the knowledge required to practice good preventive medicine that is required under new value-based care payment mechanisms. The medical curriculum has not emphasized preventive sciences such as nutrition, public health, and even a great deal of depth in genetics that will be necessary for precision medicine. This means that many physicians will need to learn new skills and also work with new stakeholders. There is also the contextual knowledge that a physician has of a single patient that needs to be taken into consideration with the community, region or group-based knowledge. It is the questions they ask, the data they focus on, the irregularities they observe, the decision process they follow, and the calculated steps they take to analyze, hypothesize, test, diagnose, and recommend a treatment. Such knowledge will distinguish a good doctor from an average one. Accessing good doctors means better care. However, the best doctor in every field cannot treat each one of us. We need a practical solution.

Corporations and factories when faced with a similar problem solve it by automating processes. If they cannot automate all the actions, they will do their best to automate most of it and scale with providing assistants to the experts. As much as we would love to duplicate this in medicine, we cannot. We can, however, provide tools and platforms for physicians to help them scale and share their skills and knowledge to everyone.

Communications and the Internet
In the twenty-first century, we have acquired more knowledge and tools than in any other time in our human history. For example, in 2012 [4, 5], 39 % of the world population had Internet access (31 % in the developing world and 77 % in the developed world). These grew from 30 % global, 21 % developing world, and 67 % developed world percentage of Internet users in 2010. This means more access to information, knowledge, and more means to communicate with each other. Figure 11.1 shows the Internet users percentage of each country's population.

Affordable personal smart devices
Another important factor is access to mobile devices and in particular, smartphones. Since the introduction of Android devices in 2008, quite a bit has been done to make smartphones affordable to many people worldwide. It is safe to assume that a medical doctor in most countries can afford an Android device (Fig. 11.2).

Free services to read and learn
Anticipating this trend, Yves Maitre d'Amato, Executive Vice President of Connected Objects and Partnerships at Orange, a global mobile operator, challenged device makers and his company to provide access to Wikipedia to African countries. Such initiatives provide access to knowledge and up-to-date information that could not have been done before. Moreover, it is cheaper than building libraries in towns and continuous spending to keep the books and journals up to date.

Wikipedia is a great human achievement. It is the first mass-used crowdsourcing free service. What is remarkable about Wikipedia is that it is built to be a free of charge service. This means anyone, regardless of income, can access this database of knowledge.[1] It is amazing to see the effort many topic-experts have made, to publish and review information using simple straightforward rules. The debate about the accuracy of each point is documented and is accessible to all of us. Peer reviews, peer pressure, collective reading and editing, and individual donations

---

[1] We do acknowledge that you need access to Internet, which is not free. However, as we have argued earlier, access to Internet is spreading fast. At some point, most of us will have access to Internet and access to this amazing library.

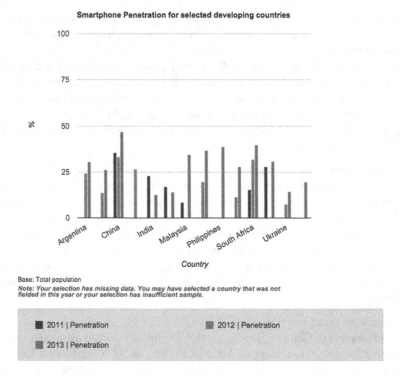

Fig. 11.2 Smartphone penetration as percentage of the population for number of developing countries [2]

made Wikipedia a great, high quality, affordable, and accessible alternative to classic textbooks and encyclopedia.

Wikipedia is a free service funded by all of us and independent of business that may influence information. This is critical for services that provide scientific facts and knowledge. It would be weird to say that the definition of diabetes is brought to you by a candy company. This will impact the credibility of the information.

Such tools are wonderful; however, they are not suitable for healthcare as is. Anyone can change part of a Wikipedia page. This will not be corrected until another person spots it. This is a problem when adopting the Wikipedia approach to healthcare. We need another step in the process: expert certification.

There are important healthcare information services that are accessible to medical professionals. They are peer-reviewed and verified. An example of such a service is UpToDate, a Wolters Kluwer service. The main issue with such a service is that it is expensive especially for medical professionals operating in low-income communities. To their credit, UpToDate does provide discounted rates for people who need it.

We do believe there is a need for a new healthcare Wikipedia that is comprehensive, peer-reviewed, free, and accessible to everyone. New paradigms where doctors can publish their research, get immediate reviews, and communicate results in Internet speed. Crowdsourcing tools can provide such a vehicle.

Successful Medical Professional Products[2]

Table 11.1 shows four different medical professionals platforms and services designed to help doctors. The differences between the four services are in the focus and in the revenue model. Doximity (doximity.com) is a service that verifies credentials of its users. Doximity also provides its users with tools to improve their career prospects and knowledge. Some may argue that Doximity is equivalent to LinkedIn. However, this is not a good comparison. With Doximity, you know that the person you are talking to is a doctor. You know where they graduated from, where they are practicing, and the status of their licenses. The Doximity team worked hard to ensure that their data is as accurate as possible. This is not the case for LinkedIn. This is a substantial difference. We cannot trust the medical opinion of someone whose identity cannot be verified. However, we can rely on the opinion of a surgeon whose identity is verified by Doximity.

Sermo (sermo.com) is one of the pioneers in medical discussion platforms. Their focus is on question and answer sessions. Their application makes it easy to snap a picture and ask a question. It is not designed for involved clinical care. However, it serves a good purpose: quick questions and answers from a specialist. It is very close in concept to Quora or Twitter: Ask a brief question and get an answer as soon as the Sermo team and community responds.

QuantiaMD provides a more sophisticated approach to medical information sharing. They provide doctors with tools to produce high-quality topic-specific or question-specific presentation. It is the equivalent of expert YouTube for medical professionals or Khan Academy. QuantiaMD team reviews and suggests topics. Doctors create presentations and videos for professional education. The outcome is equivalent to building high-quality medical textbooks. QuantiaMD is the publisher and medical professionals are the authors of high-quality media chapters organized by the QuantiaMD team. This platform is excellent for continuous medical education as well as teaching medical students.

Tabeeb's focus is on providing a platform for medical professionals to have live discussions about real-life clinical cases. It builds on crowdsourcing techniques and adapts them to the medical field. Doctors can work with their colleagues on challenging cases, share discoveries, and recommend clinical practices all within a HIPAA-compliant environment. Tabeeb includes easy-to-use imaging and video commenting tools, enabling a very interactive exchange. Tabeeb pays particular

---

[2]Please note that the author of the chapter is the founder of Tabeeb.

Table 11.1 Summary of four online medical professional only discussion services

Item	Tabeeb	Doximity	QuantiaMD	Sermo
Focus	Clinical case discussions and practice guidelines	Medical professional career growth tools and management	Continuous medical education	Doctor networking
Strength	Clinical discussions. Clinical and media tools	Verifying the identity and expertise of members	High-quality presentations	Question and answer paradigm
Revenue	Subscriptions	Professional placement companies pay to recruit doctors	Sponsored presentations	Revenue from non-medical professionals asking questions

attention to doctors working in impoverished and challenging environments. Specialists can work with them to diagnose cases, provide suggestions for treatment, and follow up with them on the progress of the patient.

Tabeeb's objective is for highly skilled specialists to share their experience with colleagues globally. They can work with them to diagnose cases, provide suggestions for treatment, and follow up with them on the progress of the patient. One way of looking at Tabeeb is that it is the evolution of telemedicine into the twenty-first century communications, i.e., social networking and media collaboration tools. Physicians can post cases, solicit opinions, discuss with experts and colleagues, share progress, and provide feedback. It is working together as a community using state-of-the-art tools.

Where Are We Headed?

The future is bright for medical professionals. They will have tools and platforms that their teachers did not have. Their influence and positive impact will be larger than all their predecessors'. We will all benefit from the new healthcare revolution. To achieve our goals of equity and high-quality care, sharing medical knowledge is critical. For that to be successful, we need the private sector to continue innovating. We also need to mature and expand the current successful platforms. In particular:

- Global Medical Professional Verification System. Doximity has been a great success. We need to see this growth to include medical professionals all over the world. The more successful Doximity is, the more the confidence we will have in the medical opinions shared in all medical platforms. Sermo has a database that includes professionals outside the USA. If Sermo's database reaches the same quality as that of Doximity and if it becomes more open, Sermo will help our cause of access to high-quality medical knowledge.

- Virtual Clinical Discussions. High-quality care cannot be achieved if the experts do not engage with their colleagues. Equity in care cannot be achieved if the person administering the medical care cannot access state-of-the-art practices and knowledge. Platforms like Tabeeb are important to providing best care to anyone anywhere. Moreover, Tabeeb can disseminate new standards for care as they emerge. Currently, it takes a long time for new standards to be communicated to medical professionals, thus impacting quality of care.
- Improved and accessible medical books are fundamental to train for the best medical professionals. QuantiaMD efforts are of great value. Medical schools will benefit from accessing this database. Please note that there are services as in UpToDate, which provides access to journals and traditional publications.

It takes much less effort to achieve our goal of quality equitable care, if we can authenticate every medical professional and provide them with an access to state of the medical knowledge and experience. It is important that such services be affordable to medical professionals in order for them to access the information and use it in their practices. We believe innovative Internet-based business models will enable such services and empower medical professionals. As mentioned above, it is also critical to draft new "Terms of Use and Service" agreements to cover doctors when they participate in such activities.

A media communication and exchange tool, such as Tabeeb, is critical in extending the reach of doctors and experts outside their local communities.

Summary

Doctors and their medical team are a critical factor to providing high-quality care and as such, need the best tools at their disposal to effectively care for their patients. Extending a doctor's reach is essential in providing equitable care.

Verified medical expert identity system + Expert crowdsourcing and communication platform + medical Wikipedia, as defined by the combination of Tabeeb + Doximity + QuantiaMD + UpToDate, will define our next generation of healthcare.

Works Cited

1. Douglas PS. ACCF/ASE/AHA/ASNC/HFSA/HRS/SCAI/SCCM/SCCT/SCMR 2011 appropriate use criteria for echocardiography. J Am Soc Echocardiogr. 2011;24.
2. Google. Our Mobile Planet. 2014. www.think.withgoogle.com/mobileplanet.en . Google.
3. GSMA. The Mobile Economy 2015. GSMA.
4. ITU. Key ICT Indicators for developed and developing countries and the world (totals and penetration rates). Geneva, Switzerland: International Telecommunications Unions (ITU); 2013.
5. ITU. Percentage of Individuals using the Internet 2000-2012. Geneva, Switzerland: International Telecommunications Unions (ITU); 2013.
6. Merriam Webster. Merriam Webster dictionary. Encyclopedia Britianica Company; 2014.

7. Odgen J. Internet penetration world map. 2014. wikimedia.org.
8. Paul F, Weigel JL, Clinton B. To repair the world: paul farmer speaks to the next generation (California series in public anthropology). California: University of California Press Books; 2013.
9. United Nations. The university declaration of human rights. United Nation; 2014.
10. Wikipedia. Appropriate use criteria (AUC). Wikimedia; 2014.

Index

Printed in the United States
By Bookmasters